THE DETOXING OF CAREGIVERS

11/10/16

Dear Laura —
We walk this path together.
Many thanks —
Regards,

Harry

THE DETOXING OF CAREGIVERS

Key Tips for Survival, Strength and Patience

L.T. Force PhD

Gerontologist

ISBN-13: 9781523356904
ISBN-10: 1523356901
Library of Congress Control Number: 2016915477
CreateSpace Independent Publishing Platform
North Charleston, South Carolina

Dedication

To all who came willingly, reluctantly, proudly, angrily, pessimistically, optimistically, frustrated, devastated, overwhelmed, and responsibly to stand by one in need—this book is a tribute to you. To all who will follow in our footsteps—we understand how you will feel.

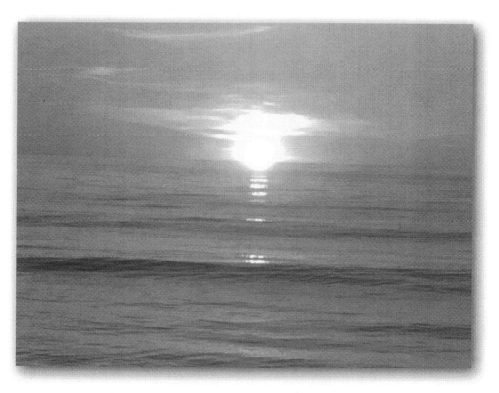

"As does the sun…you too will rise to meet the day."

Sunrise at Nauset Beach on Cape Cod, Massachusetts

(L. T. Force, PhD)

Contents

Acknowledgments

To my family, friends, teachers, mentors, and students—
you all have helped shape the way.

Introduction and Overview

Act like you matter...because you do!

(L. T. FORCE, PHD)

I bring to the discussion at this "caregiver table" a perspective derived and shaped from the experience as a son, the knowledge of a student, and the wisdom of combining both. My voice and vision in this field is influenced by real-life applied experiences in combination with theoretical knowledge and research-based exploration. With *The Detoxing of Caregivers: Key Tips for Survival, Strength, and Patience,* my intent is to not only identify the problems and concerns of caregiving but also to explore and share strategies to help.

Caregiving has become an inherent component of adult development. What was once an occasional responsibility experienced by a small number of individuals has now blossomed into a shared responsibility of millions of adults—and a predictable developmental event of adulthood. In fact, you shouldn't be surprised if you are called to take up the caregiver role. Rather, you should be surprised if you aren't. What was once an outlier, something that happens once in a while, in a certain life stage is now a predictable part of the developmental lifespan. Today, it is estimated that over 43 million adults have assumed the role of caregiver.

Overview:

- People are living longer.

- In 1900, the average life expectancy for males was 44 years of age, for females 47 years of age.

- In 1990, the average life expectancy for males was 77 years of age, for females 79 years of age. Today, life expectancy is even greater.

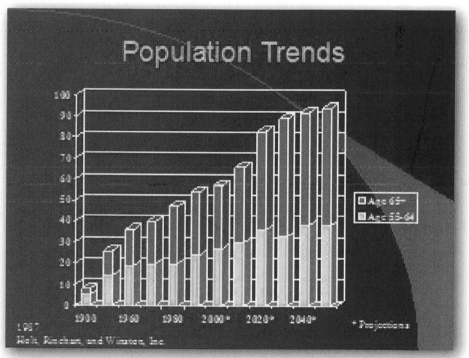

Populations Trends highlighting the increase in longevity across time

Overview

Everyday in the United States, 10,000 people turn age 65, with the fastest growing part of the population being age 100 and above.

The impact of the increase in longevity can be felt in systems and programs across our nation.

My interest has been in the field of aging for a long time—for over thirty-five years, in fact. My first clinical and administrative position was director of a medical adult day care program for a large medical center in the metropolitan New York region. The focus of my responsibility was to oversee a staff providing care to individuals with Alzheimer's disease. It was 1979, and insurance wasn't covering participation for these individuals. It was a private-pay arrangement; therefore, most individuals attending the program had the necessary resources to meet the daily rate. Individuals in the program consisted of high-level executives; members of the movie and film industry; renowned members of the medical, psychiatric, and legal arenas; and independent businessmen and businesswomen. However, it wasn't my first exposure to older individuals or the families that cared for them. More regarding this point later.

After two years of a long commute to this medical center, I secured a position closer to home in the public sector as a psychologist in a state-run institution for individuals with intellectual disabilities and psychiatric disorders.

When I accepted this position there were clinical openings in the children, adolescent, and adult units. Because of my work in the field of Alzheimer's disease, it was a natural choice that I choose the adult unit. Although it was not my first exposure to older individuals or the families that cared for them, this scenario of family caring for older adults was very close to home. In fact, it was in my own home. Nana, my father's mother and my grandmother, lived with us from the time she became a widow in her early sixties. Prior to my grandfather dying, we had moved to a different state. After his death, it was a given that Nana would move in with us. It was the thing to do during that time.

Growing up I was exposed to the presence and language of older adults. I am the youngest of three boys. My brothers were ten and twelve years older than me, and my mother and father both worked full-time, so it was Nana and me (and her friends).

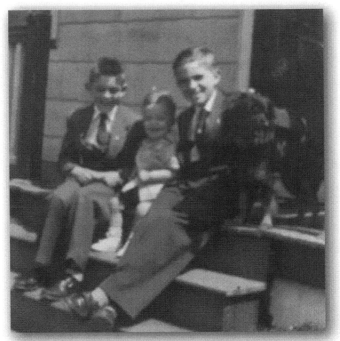

My brother Bob, me, my brother Vincent, and Blackie

We lived on the first floor of a very large apartment building in an urban center close to New York City. This apartment building housed a significant number of older and retired adults. Being one of the youngest residents and the paper boy who delivered the local daily paper, I was continually hired to do chores, walk dogs, and go to the store for a number of these older adults. What I realize today is that a number of these individuals were grateful for the support. However, I think they enjoyed my presence even more because for some of the elderly residents in the apartment building, I was the only one having a connection and a conversation with them. Strangely enough, the superintendent of the building, for years, called me "Professor." His statement became a reality.

RESEARCH

When I was completing my doctoral studies, I needed to pick a topic of focus. My first interest was the business of aging. What I was interested in was the impact that aging has on corporations; that is, how many workers were caregivers, how many workers left the corporation due to caregiving responsibilities, and what type of caregiver-assistance programs did the corporation have available for employees. When I started my research by conducting extensive literature reviews, I found that approximately 28 percent of the workforce nationwide was providing care to a family member, over 11 percent of workers (usually women) a year were resigning from their jobs as a result of competing needs, and there were a variety of models for caregiver-assistance programs being implemented across the nation in corporations. For example, there were lunchtime brown-bag seminars, in which corporations would bring in speakers with connections to different agencies such as representatives from local Area on Aging Agencies (AAAs), staff members from the Alzheimer's Association, or geriatric case managers that had a knowledge base of the services and resources within the aging network.

While all of this was interesting and worthy of further study, a soft voice in my head reminded me of two things: (1) "Focus on what you know" and (2) "You presently don't have significant contacts in corporate America." As that voice became louder and more reality based, I decided to turn my research attention to the world of adult day care, as it was termed at that point, now referenced as adult day health services (ADHS). But now the question was "What part of that arena would I study?"

THE IMPACT OF KINSHIP

With the support of my doctoral studies chairperson, Dr. Sheldon Tobin, I centered my study on the "Impact of Kinship on Accessing Social Model Adult Day Care." My doctoral studies compared the caregiving styles of spouses versus adult children, particularly in regard to their access to adult day care services. There was a specific focus on the differences among husbands, wives, and daughters in accessing this care. Adult sons were omitted from the study because I believed I would have difficulty finding a sample size of adult sons caring for their parents. In hindsight, this was a false assumption. Because as I fast-forwarded in my own life, I met a number of adult sons caring for aging parents, including my brother and myself.

As my research study continued, I started to recognize a distinct pattern difference among husbands, wives, and adult daughters as caregivers. For husbands, accessing formal outside care seemed to be initiated once they themselves could no longer drive. Husbands were asked to define "What is caregiving? and "When did the caregiving role start for you?" Their answers focused on their role in providing transportation to and from doctor appointments or to the store. Interestingly, when those two same questions were asked of older wives, *they* didn't perceive themselves as caregivers. For many, the answers surrounded two main themes: (1) "I have always been doing these tasks—cooking dinner, cleaning the house, and so on—for my family and husband" and (2) "I really don't see myself as a caregiver. I am his wife." The responses to the same two questions from caregiving adult daughters were very different. They were asked "What is caregiving?" and "When did it start?" They could almost tell you with exact precision where they were, what time of the day it was, and what they were wearing when they found out that they were going to be caregivers. It was a stark moment and a shock to the rhythm of their own lifestyle.

"Caregiving? Guilt is part of the process...as is anger and pride."

(L.T. Force, PhD)

Another variable that was explored in the study was the role of burden. Interestingly enough and based upon findings within the study, wives didn't report on either quantitative or qualitative measurement scales a sense of burden, because of their lifelong involvement in providing care to their husbands. But when husbands spoke of the onset of their burden, it was enmeshed with the inability to drive as evidence of their decline in the caregiving role. Adult daughters, however, referenced the burden of caregiving almost from the onset of the role.

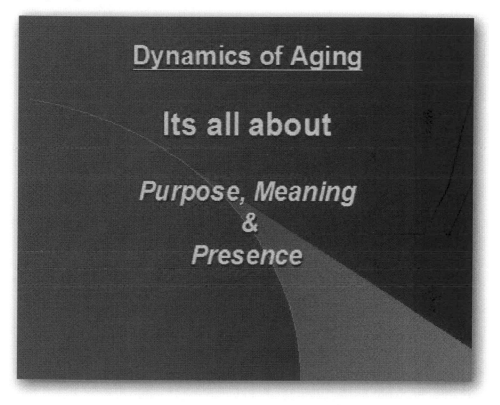

2

The Personal Side of Caregiving

BEYOND THE PROFESSIONAL AND RESEARCH SIDE OF CAREGIVING

As I mentioned, Nana lived with us. She was a tremendous presence in my life. Around the age of seventy-three, she became ill. The ultimate outcome of the diagnosis was ovarian cancer. During the time when her health was declining, our family surrounded her with love, presence, and care. My mother, who was working full-time, took a leave of absence from her job. Remember, this was her mother-in-law, not her mother. Nana's care became more involved as time progressed, and during that nine-month period, the pain elevated as did the use of morphine. Eventually, it got to the point that hospice care was required.

As in most families during times of significant illness, a pattern of communication arises. The family knew that Nana had cancer and didn't want to share that news with her. She knew that she had cancer and didn't want to tell us. The ritualistic dance of denial is not uncommon in family systems. It is a way for family members to shield the discomfort of worry and concerns. In many ways it's a dance of love. Also, one needs to remember two things. The first to remember is that at the time of her illness, circa 1968, the topic of cancer was still considered to be taboo, and it was discussed with uncertainty and a tone of secrecy. I remember as a child that a friend of my parents was diagnosed with cancer. When this man and his wife came to visit, it was recommended

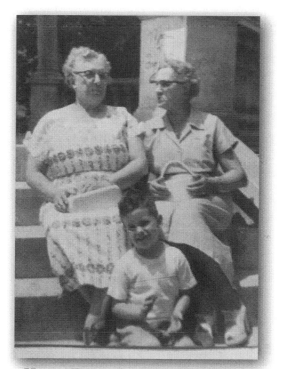

Harriet Force, a.k.a. Nana (on left), her
dear friend Frances Goheen, and me

that we not touch him because he might be contagious. As you can see, the discussion about cancer had an early primitive stage, just as the discussion about AIDS had. The second thing to remember is at this point in time the work of Elisabeth Kübler-Ross, highlighting the need and value for open discussion regarding death and dying, was just starting to be explored as a field.

In February of 1969, Nana entered Rosary Hill, a hospice center run by the Dominican Sisters. This residential hospice was approximately twenty miles from our home. In continuing our ritualistic dance of denial, we told Nana that we had to use this "hospital" because our local community hospital was full. That was not true. Twenty-two days later, March 16, 1969, Nana died.

ROSARY HILL HOME

Rosary Hill hospice was (and still is) a wonderful place committed to the care of patients and their family members. The hospice, in Hawthorne, New York, was started in Rosary Hill Home, owned and operated by the Dominican Sisters of Hawthorne since 1901. As stated on their website, "Rosary Hill is committed to providing loving, one-on-one palliative care to those suffering from terminal cancer in meeting the physical, emotional, spiritual, and recreational needs of the patients and their families." When Nana died there in 1969, little did I know that I would be back standing in the hallways of Rosary Hill five years later, in 1974.

DAD

In the spring of 1974, I was finishing my senior year of college. As a psychology major, I needed to complete an internship. I thought, "What better place to complete an internship than Rosary Hill." Having just read the Kübler-Ross book, *On Death and Dying*, I arrived for my placement interview. I was introduced to the chaplain. The chaplain was an elderly Catholic priest who was performing his ministry at Rosary Hill. During our conversation, I asked him, "Father, what would you say to a patient that asked you if he or she were dying?"

His response was, "I would tell that person to pray."

The Kübler-Ross book emphasized the importance of having open and honest dialogue with the dying patient, so I asked the elderly priest again: "Father, what would you say to a patient that asked you if he or she were dying?"

His response was, "I would tell that person to pray." This was the standard answer at Rosary Hill; at that time, they did not focus on death. Although the field as a whole was now changing its view of talking openly with the patient about the dying process, the exchanges with dying patients at Rosary Hill were not open. My internship began the next week.

In working at Rosary Hill as a student intern, I was exposed to the daily routine of a hospice. However, I was also clearly instructed to not speak to any of the patients about dying. As I became familiar with the setting, I would see some of the same patients there on my weekly visit. On average, most patients stay in a hospice for approximately thirty to forty-five days. However, there was one patient who had been residing there for ten years. This woman was a retired nurse with cancer of the spine. I always felt the staff of the hospice program allowed this nurse to stay longer as a result of professional courtesy. Ruth (a pseudonym) was a sixty-seven-year-old retired nurse. Although she was bedridden, her room was right by the nurses' station, and she was very alert regarding the comings and goings on the unit. One day while I was passing her room, she gestured for me to come over to her bedside. She said, "You're the student that is studying death and the dying. I'm sure you want to know how people feel knowing they are dying?" The only problem here, she said, was that they don't want people to talk about dying. It's almost a hidden topic. She continued, "You know that priest you met at the initial interview? Well, he has cancer too; they're just not telling him." I remember feeling that I was in the land of the body snatchers. Regardless of how I felt at that time as an inexperienced and untrained clinician, I must tell you that the warmth, care, presence, concern, and commitment from the staff at Rosary Hill Home overshadowed any and all philosophical debate about engaging or not engaging in an exchange with the dying person about the realities of dying.

As I was working on my internship surrounded by people that were in the last stage of life, my fifty-five-year-old father, John Vincent Force, died on March 6, 1974. Dad had had periodic heart attacks from the time I was in eighth grade. He was a great guy—funny, loving—and he was a man who loved his children. He died two days before my mother's birthday and was buried on her fifty-sixth birthday. This was three months before I graduated from college. The loss of my father, the symbolism of his death, and the immersion into the dying experience that I was having while completing my internship at Rosary Hill—these things made up what will always be an immense and profound part of my life.

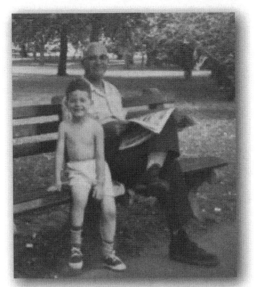

John Vincent Force, a.k.a. Dad, and me

MOM

My mother, Margaret Louise Force, died in 2015 at the age of ninety-seven. She never remarried after the death of my father. At different times, she lived with my brother and his family, and with my family for two years. I think my brother and I thought that this was what we were supposed to do. Nana lived with us after our grandfather died, so Mom should move in with us after Dad died. The only issue was that times were different, and Mom wasn't Nana. With changes in my family system, my brother arranged for my mother to obtain her own apartment. I am happy to say that she then lived independently until she was ninety-two years of age.

Around the age of ninety, we started to recognize some memory loss with Mom. We made an appointment with her primary doctor, who she loved, and explained our concerns. The doctor listened to us and then escorted my mother into an examination room. Returning fifteen minutes later, the doctor said, "She doesn't have Alzheimer's disease. She knew where she lived, her own name, the name of her children, and what season it was. She was also able to count backward by seven from one hundred to zero." We thanked the doctor; all three of us left her office smiling. When my brother and I walked to the parking lot, we looked at each other and said almost in unison, "We're out of here!" Although neither one of us are neurologists, we both knew enough that the presence or absence of Alzheimer's disease is not detected by a conversation. The next week we were at a university-affiliated memory clinic specializing in Alzheimer's screening and diagnosis. When the results of the diagnostic tests—a neurological exam, brain scans, blood profiles, and neuropsychological testing—were reviewed, the diagnosis was Alzheimer's disease. But we never used those two words, Alzheimer's disease, in front of my mother.

After the diagnosis, with medications and supervised care, my mother lived on her own for two more years. In 2011, when she was ninety-two, we received a call. The fire response team had been alerted by our mother's Life Alert alarm. When they arrived they found that she had fallen into the bathtub. My brother called me with the news. I lived sixty miles away and told him I would meet him at the emergency room. On the drive down all I kept thinking is that I hope that Mom didn't break her hip, because that would be a game changer. The good news is that she didn't break her hip in the fall. The very bad news is, unfortunately and devastatingly, she broke her neck.

Her fall was in September of 2011. The next few months were a nightmare. She was in the hospital in extreme pain, heavily medicated, very confused, and ninety-two years of age. The first approach from the medical team was to avoid surgery due to her age and complications. The protocol was a neck brace, heavy pain medication, and complete bed rest. Obviously, that didn't work. She was transferred to a rehabilitation center. The staff was nice but totally unequipped to address the severity of her situation. At one point, a nurse's aide arrived at her door and informed us that she was going to provide our mother with a shower. My brother asked, "How will you do that with her in a neck brace?"

The nurse's aide answered, "I'm going to take the neck brace off." The next day we transferred out of that facility. Obviously, this treatment approach wasn't working; therefore, we had no other choice but to move forward with the surgery.

Neck and spine surgery is difficult for anyone. Neck and spine surgery for a ninety-two-year-old person with Alzheimer's disease is a nightmare—for both that person and his or her family. The surgery was done, and our mother survived the procedure. Now the long-term rehabilitation process began. She was transferred to a rehabilitation center in New York City. A Jewish religious community runs this facility; it is world-class. When we arrived on a Friday afternoon, the prayers for the welcoming of the Sabbath day were being broadcast over the loudspeaker. The staff at this center truly knew how to address the complexity of her medical situation. Rehabilitation procedures and an interdisciplinary team were immediately assigned to her. Progress in mobility was noted and tracked. Early in her recovery, still in a fugue state from the medications, she asked me where she was. I told her the name of the facility, which identified itself with its Jewish heritage. She asked me, "Does this mean I have to become Jewish?"

I told her, "No, you don't have to become Jewish to stay here." But what this innocent question highlighted for me was the importance of familiar religious symbols in the latter part of life. Our mother practiced her Catholicism with pride and a disciplined routine throughout her life. She was strongly devoted to the Virgin Mary. In the absence of these familiar symbols and rituals, she was lost. At the completion of her rehabilitation program we transferred her to a nursing home founded by a community of the Saint Cabrini Sisters.

FIRST DAY

The transport ambulance arrived at the rehabilitation center. The driver asked if he could follow me to the nursing home. I remember driving up the parkway with the ambulance carrying our mother following behind me, and my brother driving behind the ambulance. The feelings of leading a funeral procession were overwhelming. We arrived at the admissions department of the nursing home. Arrangements were made to process the paperwork and settle her in her room. I was familiar with this nursing home. I had conducted a number of staff trainings here and was always so impressed with the commitment of the staff and the quality of the overall facilities.

After we got her settled in her room, we wheeled her into the community room. As she looked around, I could tell she wasn't feeling good about these arrangements. I asked the staff about who would be a good talkative person to introduce to our mother. I then left for the long, quiet ride home. The next day when I arrived, Mom was sitting at the lunch table socializing. After she completed lunch, we moved into the atrium. She said to me, "You know a lot of people around here, don't you?" I said I did because I had conducted staff trainings there. She then said, "So I guess you put me here to die?" At that point, I would rather have been hit by a concrete block. I really didn't know how to respond except with a quick, "No, Mom we didn't put you here to die." The ride home that night was longer and quieter than the ride home the night before.

The next day when I arrived, she asked me the same question: "So you put me here to die?"

But this time, after a night of reflection, I was ready for her question. I said: "Mom, you know that it was not possible to live alone anymore. We both asked you if you wanted to come and live with our families, and you said no. Mom, we didn't put you here to die. We made arrangements so you could live." She never asked me that question again.

The literature in the field of gerontology paints a picture that a person is at his or her worst when on a waiting list for a nursing home. In addition, it is indicated that most individuals rebound after they become settled in and familiar with the new setting. I am here to give testimony that is true. Our mother flourished in this home. She became a rock star.

The staff loved her, and she loved them. Her Irish sense of humor, her ability to socialize, and her kindness overshadowed any cognitive and physical limitations. She lived fully in her new home and died four years later with peacefulness, grace, and dignity, surrounded by family and friends that loved her more than dearly.

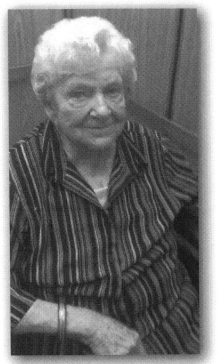

Margaret Louise Force, a.k.a.
Mom, at ninety-six years of age

"Caregiving is a long road…not a sprint…think like a marathoner."

(L.T. FORCE, PHD)

RISE AND FALL: THE TOLL OF CAREGIVING

During the last week of my mother's life, she was receiving hospice care in the nursing home. It was an emotional time, to say the least, for all of us. Hospice care started on a Monday evening after the consultation and advocacy of our dear family friend, Dr. Geri Abbatiello. My mother, a woman of strong religious conviction, would say the Rosary on a daily basis. As the pain, discomfort, and medications began to take their toll, she was unable to participate in her daily ritual. Monday evening, while we were sitting at her bedside, I noticed her rosary beads lying on her night table. I figured the best way to bring comfort to her would be to say the Rosary aloud in her presence. Monday evening, I did that, and she tried to keep up with me, but it was difficult for her. Tuesday evening, I said the Rosary aloud for her again, but she was very agitated, flailing her arms and tossing in the bed, and in discomfort. When I completed a decade on the Rosary, she would yell out, "Pray for me...Pray for me." On Wednesday and Thursday evenings, I repeated what became part of my daily routine at her bedside, reciting the Rosary aloud. However, at this point the medications had placed her in a coma-like state. On Friday, my wife and I arrived at the nursing home at 4:00 p.m. My brother Vincent had been there all day.

Around 7:00 p.m., I said to my wife, "Why don't we go and get something to eat and come back later? But I want to say the Rosaries aloud for her before we go." Sitting at her bedside, I completed the Rosary said an additional Apostles' Creed, which ends with the phrase: "I believe in the Holy Spirit, the Holy Catholic Church, the communion of Saints, the forgiveness of sins, the resurrection of the body, and life everlasting. Amen." I finished the prayer and reached over and placed my mother's Rosary beads on her night table. I turned my head toward her lying in the bed. She took two labored breaths and died.

DYING

As I tell my students in my Psychology of Death and Dying class, Hollywood and the television industry have provided us with an unrealistic portrayal of how people die. The perception that people generally go "easy into the night" is not always an accurate profile regarding the reality of the experience. My mother struggled that last week of her life. She was agitated and in pain, flailing her arms and yelling out. It was only when the heavy pain medications started to work that she became calm. The end of her life was a reflection found in the beauty of her life. To be present when she took those last two breaths after I completed her Rosaries was one of the most beautiful and powerful experiences and gifts of my life. When she did take those last two breaths, I jumped up from my chair and started to yell, "You are kidding me…you are kidding me!" I just couldn't believe how she had died. If my wife wasn't in the room, as a witness, and I came out into the hallway and told her that story, she probably would have thought, "I'm sure that's the way that you would want it to have ended, but that sounds a little exaggerated—almost like a Hollywood ending." But because she was there, she also walked away with a sense of utter awe.

After the death of our mother, we had to deal with the process and procedure associated with planning ceremonies. There were viewing services, obituary announcements, cemetery arrangements, church services, and arrangements for a place where relatives and friends who have travelled from afar could meet. And of course, we had to arrange for an Irish bagpiper for the ceremonies. All of this could be both overwhelming and at the same time a wonderful distraction from focusing on the pain of grief and loss. To our benefit, our mother had made a majority of these arrangements in her eighties when she completed a preplanning process.

GRIEVING

My cousin Billy died from a casualty suffered in the Vietnam War. My uncle immediately went out and purchased a new Cadillac. A widow from the 9/11 attacks on the World Trade Center remarried in December of 2001. The local New York tabloids profiled her actions with disdain and disgust. A dear friend of mine, when talking about the loss of her own mother, said, "The way that I handle her absence in my life is that I think of her as living in Florida, and that's why I don't see her. For me, it's because she's in Florida, not because she's dead." My friend continued with a profound statement: "They just weren't suppose to leave." Again, as I tell my students, people live uniquely, people die uniquely, and people grieve uniquely. What I have come to realize is that I will never get over the loss of my mother. I'm just trying to develop strategies on how to live alongside that loss.

LIVING

After the death of my mother, my family and I possessed a collective sense of loss and grief. However, the one thing that was consistently referenced is, "Mom would not have wanted us to be sad. She was our constant and consistent cheerleader, always looking for the bright side of life." As life continued on, we held on to that statement. What I also realized pretty quickly was that although my mother had died, I was not out of the caregiving stadium. My wife has two aging parents who live ninety miles away and have significant health needs. My take on it is that she was there for me, and I will be there for her. However, what is also clear is that providing care and presence for a parent is quite different than providing care and presence to an in-law. With my mother, my brother and I were the main "voice." With my in-laws, the final decision making is with my wife and her sister. Although I may make recommendations, it is they who take the lead in navigating this journey. And each caregiving relationship is unique to each individual and family member.

A few weeks after our mother's funeral services, we sent this letter to the administrator of the nursing home. You will note by our words how much we valued the role and presence of the Saint Cabrini's staff members. As you can see, we were blessed.

Dear Pat:

I am sure that you have heard it all. As a provider of health care, I can imagine that families have come to your door with messages of thanks and messages of concern.

Our mother, Margaret Louise Force, came to Saint Cabrini's in November 2011. Two weeks ago, at the age of ninety-seven, she passed away peacefully. We want you to know that the care, concern, and love that our mother and our family received at Saint Cabrini's goes beyond words.

In 2011, it was Lois Cartica who recommended and then advocated that we explore options at Saint Cabrini's. It was Lois who was instrumental in guiding us with compassion and care during that uncertain time. We will be forever indebted for her friendship and wisdom.

Our mother lived on 3 North. We can't emphasize enough how the care of the staff and their concern and presence combined to provide our mother with a new life. It is because of the work of all of the individuals on 3 North, representing all disciplines, that our mother was able to not only live but also create a purposeful life in the last years of her life. Whether she was engaged in recreational activities, playing bingo, attending church, going to the beauty parlor, or saying her daily Rosary in the atrium, she knew she was safe, cared for, and loved. But it was beyond the daily activity that kept our mother alive. It was the staff on 3 North that kept her alive.

You see, on a daily basis she was dressed, and washed, and fed, and transported, and provided a sense of privacy and dignity by the staff on 3 North. The staff never looked at our mother as a resident on the third floor; they knew her as "Louise" or "Margaret," a person with interests, a person with a history, and a person with a caring family. The staff treated all of us with such a sense of care, dignity, and kindness.

Our story is just one story of many. But we want to go on record. The nursing assistants, nursing staff, nursing supervisors, physician, staff members from dietary, members of the maintenance staff, and administrative support team collectively combined to create a rich and deep presence of care. We want you to know that we will be forever indebted to the women and men of St. Cabrini's.

We would hope that our words capture the depth of our feelings. We will never forget the power, presence, and quality of care that was provided by the Saint Cabrini's staff.

On behalf of the Force family, my brother Vincent and I ask that you please accept our gratitude.

Sincerely,

Lawrence T. Force, Ph.D.

Lawrence T. Force, PhD

3

How Did It Start?

Caring for yourself is not selfish…it is smart and vital.

(L. T. FORCE, PHD)

HOW DID THIS BOOK START?

In late December 2015 my wife and I made plans to go to Florida for a few days. Although she was actively addressing the health concerns of her parents, her sister would be available; we intentionally consolidated the trip into three nights and four days. We knew it would be great to get away. The thought of warmth and sun and relaxation was very inviting. As you will see in the passage below, it was further evidence of the old axiom, "Man plans…God laughs."

12/28/15

Detoxing Caregivers: The Connection with Addictions

It's Monday evening at 7:30 p.m. We were scheduled to be on our way to JFK International Airport to stay overnight at the local Marriott hotel for an early morning flight to Florida. We were truly looking forward to this five-day escape, but instead I am sitting in a Starbucks, ninety miles away from New York City.

My wife's parents live on Long Island. My father-in-law is ninety, and my mother-in-law is eighty-five. They have lived in the same house for over sixty years. About three years ago, we noticed the beginning of a downward spiral regarding health and independence. Over the last year that downward trajectory has accelerated.

Since Christmas Day, my wife has been staying at her parents' house with her sister. My father-in-law is not in a good state; his health is not good. As we were talking this morning about what we should do regarding our planned trip, it became clear early in our discussion that although we were both very much looking forward to the respite, cancelling the trip was the "right thing to do."

This has not been our first exposure to caregiving; therefore, we know about the reality of cancelling plans. In October of that year, my ninety-seven-year-old mother had passed away. She was a little Irish gal who was diagnosed with Alzheimer's disease at the age of ninety-two. Until the end of her life, she recognized us, engaged with us, and loved us.

Yesterday at the gym I was listening to an audio book on the benefits of blogging. Obviously the first recommendation is "to have something to say or add." I have a small private practice with a focus on adult development. I started to think of my research interests in aging, Alzheimer's disease, and addictions. I also started to think about the exhausted, frustrated, trapped, angry, sad, bitter, and scared adults that I have seen in my office. Some of those individuals are addressing marital problems or career roadblocks. Some of the individuals are addressing health issues or concerns about raising adult children. However, the people that I see the most in my practice are the adult caregivers of parents, or individuals and their family members that are wrestling with the wrath of addictions. As I thought more about these two groups, I realized that although they are traveling different avenues, there are a number of crossroads or similarities that they definitely share.

For adults addressing patterns of addiction, they typically are resistant and/or worn down in addition to being exhausted, scared, overwhelmed, and unsure of the future. In the addiction field, there is an emphasis on first admitting there is a problem and then addressing it through treatment—for example, detoxing, rehabilitation, and joining a fellowship/support network for follow-up, care, and recovery.

The adult caregivers for aging parents presenting themselves in my practice are also resistant and/or worn down in addition to being exhausted, scared, overwhelmed, and unsure of the future. And then I thought, "Wouldn't it be great if adult caregivers had treatment options that included 'detoxing,' rehabilitation, and joining a fellowship/support network for follow-up, care, and recovery?"

So that is what I am advocating for: the "detoxing" of caregivers. As practitioners, program developers, and policy makers we need to take the lead in creating new frontiers and creative solution-based opportunities to provide presence and care for the struggling caregiver. And if you have ever held this role, you know that all caregivers struggle. As advocates, we need to do this for my wife, her sister, and the millions of family members that have joined a club they never wanted to be a member of.

Not going to Florida was the right move.

—L. T. Force, PhD

FOLLOW-UP

Five months later, in May 2016, my father-in-law died. In the last week of his life, he was moved to a residential hospice; his death was peaceful and dignified. With both my mother and father-in-law, I was present as they crossed the threshold into eternal life. As I tell my students, I am a strong believer in the trajectory of life: "a beginning...a middle...and a new beginning."

As you can see, I have experienced caregiving from a variety of roles and perspectives: administrator, clinician, researcher, professor, son, and son-in-law. Although these different landscapes provide a distinct view, they share a similar parallel image; that is, caregiving is work, caregiving is exhausting, caregiving is powerful, caregiving is resentment, caregiving is love, caregiving can weaken you, caregiving can strengthen you, caregiving can build resiliency, caregiving is experienced uniquely, and caregiving is a part of your life you will never forget. The purpose of this book, *The Detoxing of Caregivers: Key Tips for Survival, Strength, and Patience*, is to provide reality-based tips, suggestions, strategies, and resources to help you in this role, as you are caring for someone, and to help you never forget the most important person you have to care for is you!

4

It's All about You

Regardless of the circumstances, "without you, there is no them."

(L. T. Force, PhD)

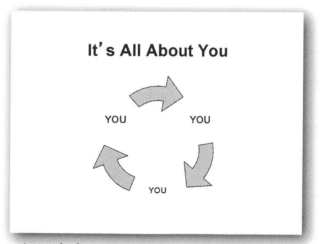

A simple diagram with a very powerful message

As the above diagram indicates, *it is all about you.*

You cannot take care of someone else or be present for someone else if you aren't taking care of yourself. In essence, the first person you are being a caregiver for is you!

NOTES/THOUGHTS/REFLECTIONS/ACTIONS

5

Different Styles of Caregiving

HEROES, MARTYRS, SNAKES, AND THE DEVASTATED

About fifteen years ago, I wrote an essay on the different caregiving styles that I found within family systems. What I was noticing from working with family members is that there were particular patterns or styles of care that surfaced. When I first wrote the article, I titled it "Different Styles of Family Caregiving: Heroes, Martyrs, and Snakes." What I described was the following: *Hero caregivers* are individuals who see a need to provide the care and do it. *Martyr caregivers* are individuals who see a need to provide the care and let everyone know they are doing it. *Snake caregivers* are individuals who see a need to provide the care and slither away.

As you can see from the descriptions of the various caregiving styles, the heroes and martyrs are present to provide the care, although they have different styles. However, the snakes are absent. What I realized was that there was another group I hadn't identified in the first writing. This group of caregivers was also not present. However, they weren't present because they were snakes; they weren't present because they couldn't bear to watch the demise of the person that they loved. The decline and fragility of their family member or friend was too overwhelming to witness. This group of caregivers isn't present because they are *the Devastated*. Therefore, I rewrote the article and titled it "Different Styles of Family Caregiving: Heroes, Martyrs, Snakes, and the Devastated."

Heroes, Martyrs, Snakes, and the Devastated: Styles of Caregiving
Lawrence T. Force, PhD

Alzheimer's disease is forever brutal. It robs the victims of their dignity and identity while stealing patience, understanding, and stamina from their families. In the years that I have been working with families who are caring for Alzheimer victims, it has been all too obvious that care has a tremendous, debilitating effect on the families. What I have noticed over time is a particular pattern that evolves within the family system. In fact, for years I have labeled these characteristics of caregiving behavior as *heroes*, *martyrs*, and *snakes*.

The Heroes
This group of caregivers provides care without question or a need for acknowledgment. For these individuals, the word caregiver does not refer to their jobs. They provide care in an unselfish manner because it needs to be done. They open their hearts, their homes, and their wallets and ask for little or nothing in return. They are the wives, husbands, daughters, sons, family members, and friends that walk the extra mile as the victim of this disease struggles against overwhelming odds. The one characteristic of this group is that you will not hear their burden as they move forward with direction and purpose.

The Martyrs
You will know this set of caregivers immediately, not because of what they do but because of what they say. These are the caregivers that insist that care is their responsibility. They will provide the care and let everyone know it is being done. They are able to tell you exactly where they were and what they were wearing when they began their caregiving. They are also quite in tune to

what others are doing, or more importantly, what others are not doing. Their payment is recognition covered with mountains of anger. When you come in contact with these caregivers, they let you know their plight and smother you with guilt. When you move toward them with the possibility of respite or relief, they become very territorial, letting you know they "can do it." The one characteristic of this group is their ability to promote their circumstances while refusing assistance or help. They are known for sending a double message, that is, "help me, but not now."

The Snakes

This group you will recognize by their absence. They are the first ones to tell you how things should be done but the last to do it. This is the group of caregivers that "keep in touch." On a regular or irregular basis, they will contact you by telephone or send an obligatory check in the mail. This is the group that refuses to dirty their hands. When you call them with information or an update about the patient's health status, they will be the first to tell you about the difficulty that they encountered on their last vacation, or better yet, they will lament to you about the difficulty they are experiencing while running their dog to the veterinarian's office weekly. They don't hear you because they don't want to hear you. They are deliberately missing; in fact, they are hiding. The one characteristic of this group is their absence.

The Devastated

For a number of years, I felt these were the three major categories of caregivers: heroes, martyrs, and snakes. But I also began to realize that there is a fourth group. These unnamed caregivers were also not involved, not because they did not want to be but rather because they couldn't be involved. Recently, I came to identify this group as *the devastated*. For this group of caregivers, the sight of the demise of their spouse, parent, family member, or friend afflicted with Alzheimer's disease is too devastating to handle. They are not shunning their responsibility or turning away from their obligation—they just can't deal with it. For this group of caregivers, their trademark is anguish. Knowing that they are helpless in trying to stop the Alzheimer dance as it progresses to its end, they become ravaged with despair. For them, absence is the only choice for survival.

These are examples of the four major caregiving patterns I have encountered in my clinical work. Do more patterns exist? Most definitely! Does everyone fit into a specific category? Obviously not! However, there are trends in Alzheimer's care. As the disease progresses and our ability to work with victims and families continue, other patterns will emerge. As a society and as individual practitioners, we need to be continually vigilant of new trends and models that develop within the caregiver arena. The outcome of our effort will be to help increase the quality of care provided.

As I was telling my friend Theresa Giovanniello about including "Heroes, Martyrs, Snakes, and the Devastated: Styles of Caregiving," she said, "I think there is also another group called the *wolves*. These are the caregivers that swarm in, take over, isolate the person from their family members, and take complete control." I agree. I then started to realize there was another group that I have witnessed—the *liquidators*. This group of caregivers swoops in and gains sole control of the finances. Their primary self-centered interest is with assets, even at the expense of the quality of life of the person who owns those assets. As you can see, there are multiple styles of caregiving.

DETOXING CAREGIVERS: KEY TIPS FOR SURVIVAL, STRENGTH, AND PATIENCE

Although there are different styles and strategies in caregiving, there are also some common overlapping patterns. As indicated earlier, caregiving is work, caregiving is exhaustion, caregiving is powerful, caregiving is resentment, caregiving is love, caregiving can weaken you, and caregiving can strengthen you. The question is, "Are there strategies and tips that you can incorporate into your daily life as caregiver that will help you survive, increase your strength, and increase your patience?" I say yes. Interestingly, I asked my wife this same question. She responded by saying, "I don't have time to do other things; I need to do this job." It was interesting, however, that she answered this question as she was returning from the gym, and this was just prior to us going out for a walk on the golf course with our golden retriever. My response to her and my statement to you is exactly the same: "Don't underestimate the simple things you are already doing in your life. You may say that you don't have time to exhale or relax, but you may already be doing simple things that are working to help you through this situation. A good recommendation is to take a look at what you are doing, and then let's see if those things can be enhanced and expanded."

WHAT WORKS?

Caregiving impacts every part of your being. The question is why some people can take on this role with relative ease and mastery while other individuals find it to be an emotional, psychological, financial, and spiritual assault. The answers are as unique and varied as the number of individuals that populate this world. What we do know is, as I have stated, "all behavior occurs within a family system. And when families work, they work. And when families don't work, they don't work."

QUOTES

"I despise my siblings. I feel that everyone has run for cover. The whole decision-making process has been dumped on me."

—*Daughter, age fifty-three, one of four siblings*

wasn't for my sister, I don't know what I would do. ...nd her family (husband and kids) have been a godsend for my parents."

—SON, *AGE SIXTY-ONE, ONE OF TWO SIBLINGS*

There are so many variables that impact caregiving; for example, health (of the caregiver and care receiver), wealth (of the caregiver and care receiver), distance (both geographical and emotional), perception of equity and fairness (is everyone pulling their weight with shared responsibility?), access to resources and support services (including respite and downtime), and finally, compliance, willingness, and appreciation (are the individuals who are receiving the care receptive and grateful, or are they resistive, arrogant, nasty, and unappreciative of your efforts?). The reality that often gets diluted in the process is that *caregivers have rights and feelings too*! This fact is so important to remember. Not only do you have rights and feelings but also you have a life. With the responsibility of caregiving, there are times that life gets diverted, hijacked, derailed, or put on pause.

Two weeks before my mother died, my youngest son, Patrick, said to me: "Dad, a friend of mine from work and I were talking, and I have to tell you, obviously I'm concerned about Grandma. But as I told my friend, I'm also worried about you. When Grandma dies, what are you going to do with your time?" This is such a great innocent and powerful question. It's also further evidence that caregiving becomes more than a role; it becomes such an integral part of your life, your routine, your thoughts, and your actions. It becomes *you*. And there is nobody who needs to be taken care of more than you...because without a "you" there is no "other."

EXHALE

In life, all things evolve. This is true also of clinical practice. My early training in psychology focused on the school of behaviorism. The simple orientation of this approach is that "things are learned...and therefore, things can be unlearned." As I moved on in my graduate studies, I gravitated toward the psychoanalytic school of thought. Within this paradigm, the belief centers on symbolism and interpretation of behavior; that is, things aren't as they seem. As my training and experience continued on, I found myself aligning with less theoretical-driven paradigms and more applied techniques. I found myself practicing task-centered interventions combining a cognitive-behavioral perspective. Then, in what was more than just a coincidence, I was introduced to solution-focused work. I really like this perspective; the focus is not on problems but solutions in the here and now. I must tell you I find this perspective refreshing and rewarding.

As I was moving through time in my clinical practice and training, life was moving along also. My kids were growing up, graduating high school, and moving on to college. My days of going to high school track meets and football games were on the downswing. One day as I was watching the news on TV, a reporter highlighted a story about a plane crash at JFK Airport. The reporter mentioned that the family members of the passengers on the plane were gathering at the airport and that the mental-health workers from the American Red Cross had started to arrive at the airport. With that, the reporter panned to a video of the mental-health workers arriving. I started to think that maybe I should do something like this. I had the training and experience. I also had more time now with the kids getting older and leaving high school. Later that month, I contacted the American Red Cross and became trained as a disaster mental-health specialist.

Once I received the training, my name was placed on a list. If the Red Cross responded to a disaster where mental-health workers were needed, I was called. In the first year I was called a couple of times for airplane crashes, fires, or flooding. And then, late afternoon on September 11, 2001, I received a call that would change my life.

I remember standing in my driveway, pacing, thinking, "Do I really want to go there?" And then I started to think, "This is where the rubber hits the road. This is why I completed this training and volunteered. I need to go." When I arrived at the Red Cross headquarters that evening, it was pandemonium. Lines and movement surrounded all of us. After I was processed, I was assigned to ground zero. It was everything that you have read—that is, complete chaos, despair, and valor all wrapped in one. The idea was to be present. I remember all of it.

Eleven months later on August 22, I was outside walking my golden retriever pup and told my wife I didn't feel good. I went inside, and it was like somebody had shot me in the stomach. I didn't realize as I was hitting the floor that it was the beginning of a yearlong odyssey that would change my life. I had five operations within the year, multiple hospitalizations, external drains for ten months, and a forty-pound weight loss before I got back up. Vital in my recovery were prayer, family, outstanding medical care, and my friend Geri, who came to my house one day. I was lying on the couch at 148 pounds with external drains in me, and she told me, "Get up." Get up? I couldn't even go down the driveway to get my mail. She told me, "You need to not look at your life through your medical issues. You need to disconnect your mind from your body and create the image of how you want it to be: competent, in control, healthy, strong…" She went on. That day changed my recovery. I did get up; each day I was stronger. That day, Geri's input introduced me to the power of imagery.

I resumed my life and began teaching again with a strong appreciation of the power of imagery, and Geri and I became trained as clinical hypnotherapists. I also began to integrate clinical hypnotherapy techniques into my practice. What I started to recognize almost immediately was that breathing in and out and going deeper and deeper into a more relaxed state with each breath you take truly was having a powerful influence on the lives of my clients. As they just practiced the simple act of breathing and focusing on the moment, focusing on the now, they began to make positive adjustments in their lives.

6

Fast-Forward and DSBT

I realize I have given the best part of my life…to his care.

—Sixty-eight-year-old wife and caregiver

FAST-FORWARD AND DSBT

Today, my practice continues with a focus in adult development. I see individuals who present issues with anxiety, stress, regret, doubt, and an overall sense of being overwhelmed. What I offer is a treatment intervention that I titled *dimensional solution-based treatment* (DSBT). The intervention is based upon the theory of dimensionality. The focus of the theory is that life events are the dimensions in one's life—the dimensions of health, wealth, career, children, family, and so on. The role of the therapist, from my perspective, is not to "fix" you, because you are not "broken." Rather, it's to help you incorporate other positive and adaptive patterns and interests into your life that will assist you in changing your perception of people, events, and circumstances.

The theory of dimensionality is:

$$Ph = S + D$$
$$Ph = \text{Personhood}$$
$$S = \text{Stages}$$
$$D = \text{Dimensions}$$

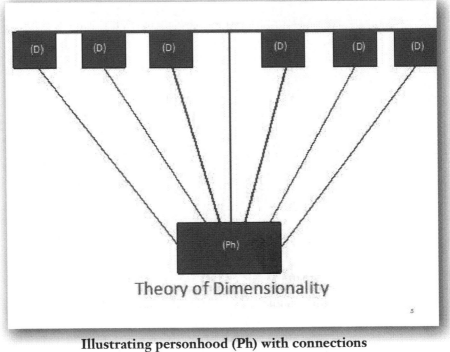

**Illustrating personhood (Ph) with connections
to the dimensions (D) within one's life**

As a therapist, I don't have the power to change the stage of development that you are in. I can't (nor can you) change your age. Nor can you or I change the complexity of the life events. However, as you integrate a new awareness into your life and as a result change the way you perceive these events, I can help you. You see, it is not changing events or others; it is helping you change you. How? My belief is beyond talk therapy. For me, from what I have witnessed, it is not just the biopsychosocial approach that is the key but rather the combination of cognitive (talk therapy and clinical hypnotherapy), energy (nutrition, wellness, and spirituality), and movement (exercise, yoga, Pilates, walking, etc.) paradigms that matters. How strongly do I believe that this matters? Today, I will only see individuals in therapy if they are working in concert with a nutritionist and engaged in a formal or semiformal exercise regime. And this is what I bring to the caregiver table: a notion that if you want change, it is only you that can spearhead that campaign.

7

Simple Steps

If you lose yourself (physically, emotionally, spiritually), everyone loses

(L. T. FORCE, PHD).

I KNOW IT'S OVERWHELMING: BREATHE IN AND BREATHE OUT

I know that sounds very simple. It is, and it's much simpler and much better than hyperventilating. The importance of focusing on your breathing is often overlooked.

Years ago, when my friend Geri and I became trained as clinical hypnotherapists, we learned about the importance of focusing on the breath. Anxiety and stress are entities that we have learned to express, feel, and live across our lifetime. The good news is that anxiety, stress, and fear can be unlearned. And the first step is to just breathe.

FACES AND PLACES

I have clients that present themselves in my practice with anxiety, stress-related fears, and ritualistic-based obsessions. As they begin to tell their story, I hear multiple references to tightness, heart palpitations, fist clenching, and racing thoughts. With a focus on breathing and a focus on the *now*, those mind-body reactions can be managed. In 2014 I attended a weeklong training on Cape Cod given by Ron Siegel. The title was Using Mindfulness Techniques as a Therapeutic Intervention. During the presentation, Dr.

Siegel stated, "In working with clients, one realizes that a function of the therapist is to help clients stay in the now." He continued, stating, "When clients focus on the past, it's all about depression. When clients focus on the future, it's all about anxiety. In helping clients focus on the now, you can help them address their anxiety and stress." That is a great statement. And it all begins with breathing in and breathing out.

EXERCISE

Lie down on a bed or couch or sit comfortably in a chair. Place your hands comfortably by your side or on your lap. Take a look at the ceiling. Begin to focus on part of the ceiling that you haven't noticed before. Continue to focus on that part of the ceiling and breathe in and breathe out. As you are breathing in and breathing out, close your eyes. Know that it is safe and comfortable, and you are in control. Continue to breathe in and breathe out. And with each breath you take, go deeper and deeper into a relaxed state. Just focus on your breathing. And if your mind starts to race, which it probably will, just continue to focus on your breathing. Breathe in and breathe out, and go deeper and deeper into a relaxed state. Exhale.

THE POWER OF IMAGERY

The focus on breathing can be very powerful. The simple act of breathing in and breathing out has long-standing proof of being effective. However, breath work in combination with the use of imagery can be doubly powerful. When Geri sat at the end of my couch, she said to me, "Get up." Little did I know then the power of those words. It was like the phoenix rising from the ashes. And when I said to Geri, "I can't even go to my mailbox at the end of my driveway," her words to me—and now my words to you—were, "You cannot look at the world through the eyeglasses of your medical condition." And in this case, it's through the eyes of your caregiving responsibilities.

VISUALIZATION

Years ago, I knew a college professor who would say, "Individuals take about eighteen months to make significant changes in their life. That is how long they think about how they want to be and then start to imbed these images into their daily practices." I found this to be an interesting statement. Years later, I was teaching a social psychology course as an adjunct professor for a community college in a maximum-security prison. During one of the lectures, I spoke about Elliot Aronson's idea of the idealized self-concept. This theoretical perspective indicates that an individual can focus on an image of how he or she ideally sees oneself and then move his or her daily practice in that direction. As I was presenting this material, a student in the class raised his hand and said, "Man, you don't get it. You're talking to us about an idealized self-concept. We're in here for life—you just don't get it." He was right. I didn't get it.

I don't necessarily believe that it takes eighteen months on average to modify one's perception of self. I also don't believe that the role of caregiving is a prison, although there are times it may feel prison-like. What I do believe is that if you want to change, then act like you want to change. "Doing the same thing over and over again and expecting different results is the definition of insanity" truly applies to the role of caregiver. If it feels overwhelming, then maybe you need to integrate things into your daily life that will help to reduce the stress. The power of breathing and visualization—although it may be outside of your comfort zone—can be a very valuable survival technique.

Try these exercises both at times when you feel stressed out and at other times when you are not feeling stressed. Try them a couple of times of day. If you don't have the opportunity to lie down or sit in a comfortable chair, just try it where you are. You can even be standing. Breathe in and breathe out, and focus on your breathing. With each breath you take, you go deeper and deeper into a relaxed state. I tell you, it clearly works.

Also remember that you are not a victim. Yes, these can be difficult, stressful, and overwhelming times. But change requires work. And if you are not feeling the way you want to or the way you think you should be feeling at this point in your life, invest in you. Want to change the situation (dimension of caregiving) immediately? Change the way you look at it. Clearly remember: I am not speaking about this from a theoretical hands-off perspective. I have been in the caregiving trenches for over seventeen years. I realized that after I wrote this sentence, it should have read, "I was in the caregiving trenches." There are times that I still can't believe that Mom has died. I realize that as of this writing it has only been three and a half months. But there are times that it feels like it has been three and a half millenniums. And at other times, I forget that she has actually died.

Breathe in and breathe out. Simple? Yes! Powerful? Yes!

Breathe in and breathe out. It will change your world.

COMPLETE SUBMERSION

If you want the full experience of enhancing relaxation and imagery, I recommend that you try the following:

- Begin the exercise in a lying or comfortable sitting position.
- Don't sabotage the experience. Try to enhance the experience by turning the phone off. If possible, dim the lights in the room.
- Add your favorite background mediation music/or soft music.
- Begin by focusing on part of the ceiling you haven't seen before.
- Breathe in and out. Relax. Inhale and exhale.
- Stay focused on your breathing.
- With each breath, go deeper and deeper into a relaxed state.
- Continue this exercise for 5 to 10 minutes…breathing in and breathing out

Although these recommendations will enhance your experience, you will find more benefit if you completely submerge yourself in the process. How best to do that? The best way is to step outside of yourself and try to perceive yourself from a distance. You know better than anyone what issues need to be addressed. You also know in your heart that *you can't take care of someone else if you can't take care of yourself.*

8

Taking Care of All of You

Caregiving itself can be an addiction. It can take over your thoughts, actions, and focus.

—BARBARA, CAREGIVER, AGE FIFTY-EIGHT

As I previously indicated, my clinical practice focuses on issues in adult development. I have had clients come to my office as they are addressing concerns of anxiety or depression. I practice short-term psychotherapy with an emphasis on the here and now.

I believe the following—and I share these principles with my clients:

- Life happens outside of the office of the therapist.
- I'm not your hero, and I can't "fix" you, because you are not "broken."
- Everybody has "stuff."
- My role is to help you identify patterns of behavior and then to help you develop strategies that decrease those patterns as you are also identifying patterns of behavior that *are* working—and to help you develop strategies to increase those behaviors.

The first session with a client is what I call the "landscape" session because I am gathering information and concerns that present a wide landscape.

I'm trying to get a sense of who is who and what is what. When the discussion of anxiety or depression comes up, I ask them a few simple questions:

- Have you had any medical work-up?
- Have you ruled in or ruled out the presence of Lyme disease? Lyme disease can present itself as depression, anxiety, and cognitive impairment (dementia).
- What about alcohol or drug use?
- How does your sleep pattern look?
- Have you had a head injury over the last ten years? A head injury can present itself as impulse disorders, anxiety, and depression.
- What does your diet look like?
- Do you incorporate any formal exercise into your daily routine?

Why do I ask these questions? Because I think they matter. I remember when I was working as a psychologist for the state of New York. In that role, I was assigned a caseload of individuals with intellectual disabilities who were living in a group home. There was a middle-aged female client who lived in one of the group homes who was presenting aberrant behavior and acting out. The group-home administrator had asked for input from the interdisciplinary treatment team (ITT), which consisted of a medical doctor, nurse, psychologist, social worker, recreational therapist, and dietician on how best to address the behavior. The ITT members assembled at the dining room table for a discussion while the client was sitting in the kitchen area of the house. The members of the ITT agreed on the recommendation to introduce a small antianxiety medication to address the outbursts. We then asked the client to join us so we could discuss our recommendation with her. When she arrived at the dining room table, a staff member asked her if she would like a cup of coffee. She said yes. As the coffee was placed on the table in front of her, the client proceeded to put six teaspoons of sugar into her coffee. Teachable moment: here we were recommending an antianxiety medication to help with her anxious behavior, and here she was loading up her coffee cup with six teaspoons of sugar.

Obviously we withdrew our recommendation for the antianxiety medication and focused on first weaning her off the sugar and caffeine. I will never forget this scenario, and it is one that I am sensitive about today as well. When clients come in today with concerns of anxiety or depression, and they tell me they are eating three bags of potato chips and drinking four Cokes or Pepsis a day, my answer is, "Hello! Maybe the initial focus needs to be on your diet and nutrition before you call in the 'psychiatric police.'" I hold the same belief system regarding the value of daily exercise and how important that is.

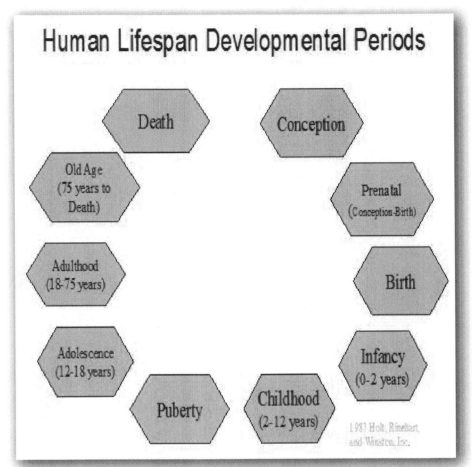

This developmental perspective was presented in a 1987 psychology textbook. Please note the ages that are assigned to the stages. For example, adulthood is age eighteen to seventy-five, and old age is age seventy-five to death. Today, those ages do not reflect these developmental stages.

NEW PERSPECTIVE ON AGING, FORCE, 2010

Re-Definition of Aging

Very Oldest-Old	100	Self-Children-Formal Support
Oldest - Old	91+	Self – Children - Peers
Old - Old	76-90	Spouse – Children - Self
Young Old	61-75	Spouse-Children-Peers-Work
Mid-life Phase 3	51-60	Spouse-Children-Parents-Peers-Work
Mid-life Phase 2	41-50	Spouse-Children-Parents-Peers-Work
Mid-life Phase 1	31-40	Spouse-Children-Parents-Peers-Work
Young Adulthood	19-30	Parent-Person- Peers-Work
Adolescent	11-18	Parent Person - Peers
Childhood	3-10	Parent – Child - Peers
Infancy	0-2	Parents - Child
Prenatal Period		

In this chart, stages are listed in the left column. In the middle column are the accompanying ages, and the column to the left identifies the dimensions that the individual is typically addressing. Please note the redefinition of aging; that is, adulthood is further defined across the ages into particular stages. As well, please note the new stage of the very oldest old, the fastest growing demographic stage today (individuals over one hundred years of age).

Note: The symbol at the top left of the chart indicates the importance of viewing age from a vertical perspective (stages) as well as a horizontal perspective (dimensions). Dimensions are the issues that the person is addressing in that particular stage.

NOTES, THOUGHTS AND REFLECTIONS:

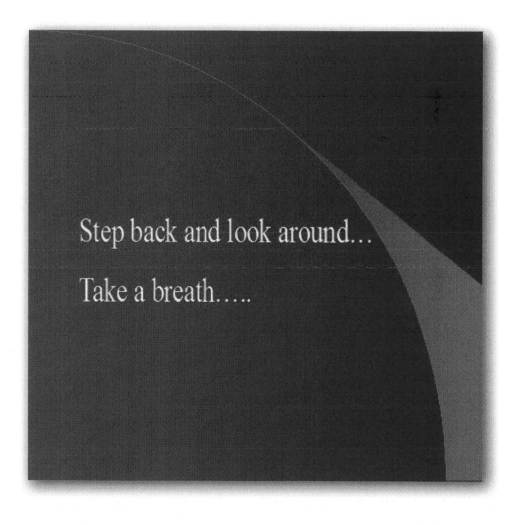

"I have two stories for your book, *The Detoxing of Caregivers: Key Tips for Survival, Strength, and Patience.*"

—*Laura Stark, public speaker; e-mail: Laura@LauraStark.net*

There is a great saying in the Alzheimer's support group I attend: don't argue with them, don't try to reason with them, and if it is not a safety issue, just let it go.

I hear this over and over each month.

While caring for my father for twelve years when I lived in Dallas and was working, I received no help from my older brother, who lived on Long Island. This is very typical.

I saw my father every Saturday and took him out to eat. When I couldn't get my own chores done, I finally asked him if it would be OK if we skipped that week's visit.

The biggest thing I learned to say to my dad was, "Dad, I could use your help." I don't know of one parent that would not want to help his or her child. I always got a yes, of course.

The other issue is my ninety-three-year-old mother-in-law. For years she told all her friends how I hung the moon. I was terrific. After her husband died, we eventually moved her from New Jersey to Denver, as there was no other family there to care for her.

Even back in New Jersey she would say, "I'm having a senior moment." Little did we know that this was a red flag of early onset dementia. Who knew she was a Jekyll and Hyde?

She eventually turned on me when the paranoia set in. She accused me of stealing everything from her. I stole some of her expensive clothes, her sterling tea set, her car, her purse, and, yes, even her toaster.

She still tells her grandchildren how I steal from her.

In my support group, I was able to share that it hurt me so much how two-faced she was to me. I told my husband and the group that I no longer want to subject myself to her, yet I know it's the disease. I have only seen her twice now.

I needed to take care of me first. She is ninety-three years old, and I am sixty-six and have a lot more living to do.

My biggest question is why do people who have this disease, in which there is no quality of life, hang on so long? I have told my husband to have a discussion with her about letting go. I did that with my father, and he chose to let go. I told him, "I will be OK. It's time to go dancing with Mom in heaven." My parents won ballroom dancing trophies.

I hope this helps you.

■　■　■

Detoxing Caregivers: A Personal Reflection
by Barbara A. Johnson

Ah, the sunroom. I never gave this room much thought. My parents added it to their house about twenty years ago, and my father spent many hours enjoying the calm quiet of its sturdy, windowed surroundings while propped up in his recliner. With heat and air conditioning and a big ceiling fan, the room could be used almost year-round in Texas, and the addition of a television with comfy recliners made it a relaxed and casual retreat to view nature or listen to the rain on the metal roof. Mom and Dad (and the family dog) would sit in matching recliners to watch their favorite programs or doze. It was Dad's favorite room in the house, and he spent many hours there when not sitting at his big wooden desk in the adjacent den.

The sunroom was always an afterthought to me, as my visits to the house were to drop my bags in the guest room as I decompressed from travel, or later, when I moved back to the area, to come for a meal or help with household tasks. During those times, I passed the sunroom to wave hello to my father in his chair as I came and went through its doors. I always admonished him to move to another part of the house during the days of a hot Texas summer, but he would creep back in once the sun had set.

After my father passed away, the sunroom sat empty except for the times when my widowed mother would sit in its bright comfort to watch television and the birds outside. My father's chair remained, and I would sit in it for a while during my visits to chat and get my "marching orders" regarding anything my mother needed help with. Again, I pretty much passed through the sunroom on my way to somewhere/something else. Mom needed no admonishment regarding the wisdom of seeking a cooler room though when the hot Texas sun required all the blinds to be closed on a summer day. Solar screens were added to reduce the effects of the sun's glaring rays, but even those couldn't keep the temperature comfortable for her. Spring and fall became the times of year when she would seek the comfort of the sunroom.

A few years have gone by; so much has changed, but that sunroom remains. Mom experienced a series of falls, which resulted in two back injuries and limited mobility. She stopped sitting in the sunroom, and it became an empty, unused furnished space. Frequent treks to the house to troubleshoot maintenance issues, get groceries, help her with ADLs (activities of daily living), and basically run her household—all while I held down a full-time job and part-time academic pursuits and lived twenty miles away—became too much for me to manage. I was exhausted, stressed, and constantly worried about what would happen next. I wasn't spending much time in my own home. The emergency response team and a key to Mom's front door for use by a dear neighbor weren't enough anymore. My cell phone was on twenty-four-hour standby, and the gas tank was always full for the increasingly frequent demands on my time.

So I moved into the family home. I sold my house in a booming suburb for top dollar, quit my job, and decided to devote my time to completing my doctoral dissertation, caring for my mother, and redirecting my efforts for the next chapter of my life. The house has been redecorated, accommodations have been made for Mom's limitations, and I'm now in charge of just one household instead of two. I've gotten to know my parents' neighbors and become involved in community affairs. I am a bigger part of a different world now.

Still have stress. Still fall into bed exhausted at the end of the day. Still frustrated by the feeling that my life is standing still due to the needs of others. There are no vacations, no hours of shopping or dining with my friends. My time has to be planned in or away from the house. At times I shed tears of frustration or find my temper flaring.

But at night, when Mom is finally comfortable in bed and I've closed up the house for the night, I eagerly settle into *my* comfy chair in the sunroom and enjoy the peaceful glow of the new television while I savor a big glass of wine to end my day. And if it's gently raining outside, the sound of the drops on the metal roof remind me that for now, this is where I need/am supposed to be. My life isn't really standing still, but I have to be still during those precious solitary late evening hours to realize that. The sunroom is my detox center, and I have come full circle with its presence. I sneak off to it whenever I can, and its welcoming embrace soothes my soul better than any support group. I whisper to Dad that I am taking care of things now, and thanks for building that sunroom twenty years ago.

■ ■ ■

THE ARTIST AND JIM

When I was completing my doctoral studies, I enrolled in a family-practice class. During the semester, it was expected that I would work with a family in their home. I chose a family that was wrestling with Alzheimer's disease. When I arrived at their home, I was introduced to Helen, the wife and caregiver, and Jim, the husband and Alzheimer's patient. Helen was seventy-nine years old, and a professional artist. Jim was eighty-two years old and had been an executive in the finance industry. Jim and Helen were the parents of two adult children who lived 250 miles away. Jim was diagnosed three years ago and was in the late stages of Alzheimer's disease. At our first in-home session it was apparent that Helen was committed, caring, and exhausted. She was the only one who was providing presence and care to Jim. During our first session we spoke about two to three "problem issues" that they would like to address. Helen spoke nonstop while Jim, stoic and quiet, sat at the table. We agreed that we would target three issues: (1) assistance with navigating the Medicare/insurance maze, (2) assistance with recommendations about programs and services that would add support for Jim and Helen, and (3) help for Helen to recapture some time in which she could practice her trade and paint on a daily basis for relaxation and respite. It sounded easy to address these three issues and to develop short-term tasks that would help relieve the stress for both Jim and Helen. However, it was far from easy. It was agreed that we would meet for a total of four sessions.

When I arrived for the second session and rang the doorbell, Jim answered. His attire was color coordinated, he was cleanly shaven, and his hair was combed. Helen was standing behind him wearing a stained sweatshirt, her hair unkempt, and looking totally overwhelmed. At first glance, if you weren't aware of who the caregiver was and who was experiencing Alzheimer's disease, you would think it was Jim as caregiver and Helen as the person struggling with Alzheimer's. It shortly became clear why Helen looked so disheveled.

During our session Helen explained that she had been awake for two days. She was not able to sleep at night because Jim would get up in the middle of the night to use the bathroom. He would walk around the bed, turn, and urinate on the bed. She also admitted that in order to deal, she had started to take the medications that the doctor had prescribed for Jim. Helen was at the end of her rope. Obviously we were at a crisis point.

There is no magic in caregiving. However, there are small steps that can bring relief. At the session, Helen was ready to reach out for outside support. We immediately accessed the local county office for the aging (AAA) and a home health-care agency. Helen agreed to have someone come into the home for Jim four days a week, five hours per day. We also agreed that during the time the home health-care aide was in the home, Helen would spend some time in her studio painting, drawing, thinking, relaxing, and…escaping. I must tell you, this assistance, though limited, was a godsend. Helen was able to recapture some semblance of what was predictable and useful in her life.

We met for two more sessions and worked our way through the Medicare/insurance maze. In four sessions, we were able to pierce a small amount of the overwhelming state that Helen and Jim were feeling. Six months later Jim passed away.

There is no magic in caregiving. There is no magic potion to completely relieve caregiving stress; however, the small steps can be giant leaps forward.

Sand Prints

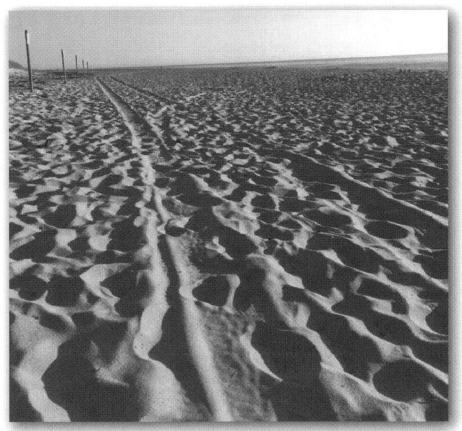

Please note the footprints…some in circles…some heading
backward…with a road straight ahead…guided by the ocean on
one side and a beach fence on the other…and never alone.

9

Holistic Triage

In the world of medicine, the term *triage* connotes what concerns will be addressed first—that is, the most pressing issue. In further developing dimensional solution-based treatment (DSBT) intervention, the question was, "What would be the best intervention strategy that could be used to address adults in distress?" This work came out of an interest and collaboration in the field of aging and addictions. What evolved from that question was the development of an intervention strategy termed *holistic triage*.

Holistic triage is an approach that provides the individual with tools and a skill set to build resiliency. Holistic triage[1] emphasizes natural supports to enhance cognitive (thinking and imagery), energy (nutrition, wellness, and spirituality), and movement (exercise, strength building, yoga, Pilates, and breath work) domains. In addition, the holistic triage paradigm places a heavy emphasis on the value of internal reflection, knowing that, as I have indicated in my practice with clients, "there is no one who speaks to us more than we speak to ourselves." And the problem is that "we say negative, derogatory, and off-putting things to ourselves that we would never allow others to say to us." Therefore, the DSBT approach encourages one to employ a self-driven therapeutic process, which can be initiated immediately and daily by altering the way we internally speak and dialogue to ourselves about who we are. Strength and hope—and therefore, the positive/supportive words that we say to ourselves—can be

---

1 Holistic triage: mind-body-spirit exercises and interventions are integrated into daily practice.

derived from periods of reflection, meditation, and prayer. This creates a spirituality connection. The source in which one finds a sense of relief, guidance, strength, and solace will be dictated, uniquely and individually, by each person.

IMPLEMENTING PRACTICE

When individuals arrive for their first appointment, they have been guided by either an internal voice or driven by an external voice (recommendations of friends, a spouse, children, a boss, or the legal system), and they need to talk to someone. As I have indicated previously, the first session is about gathering the overall picture and then drilling down to help frame out two or three problems or concerns, which I now refer to as dimensions, that they would like to focus on. For some clients, this is their first time in seeking therapeutic help. For others, they have a long history in accessing therapeutic assistance. I had one client who came to see me. She was a woman in her midthirties. She came in, was personable, and had good eye contact. After she completed the intake forms and we began the discussion, she immediately dropped her head and started to speak in a low-toned voice. I stopped her and said, "Boy, do you know how to do this. You really know how to do what you consider to be therapy—that is, head down and low voice with no eye contact. The only thing that you don't have on is your 'therapy uniform.'" As I challenged her on this observation, she began to laugh. I asked her, "How many therapists have you seen?"

She responded, "I've seen eight therapists."

I said, "Now I understand."

She continued to laugh at what I had said to her and raised her eyes and her voice.

With integrating the dimensional solution-based treatment (DSBT) and holistic-triage paradigms, I now inform clients in the first session that my form of treatment consists of a cognitive approach accompanied by clinical hypnotherapy—that is, the use of relaxation techniques and imagery—and also the recommendation that they work on the energy domain (nutrition, hydration, wellness, and spirituality) and the movement domain (exercise, walking, stretching, and meditating). In other words, as noted, "If you want to change…act like you want to change."

I also let them know that change is not about growing up—it is about growing in and growing out. And that, my friends, is my advice to you. If you want to survive this caregiving role, act like you want to survive this caregiving role by getting stronger and more patient with yourself as a caregiver and with your care receiver. You have the tools to do this.

WHAT DOESN'T WORK?

Once I said to a dear friend that she would probably benefit enormously from using a time-management program. She had always been talking about how overwhelming her life was and that she wasn't making any progress on certain projects. When I recommended that she might want to explore the use of a specific program, she told me, "I don't have time to use a time-management program." There is a definite irony in her response.

I advise you not to be like her. Take control of what can be controlled. Change what can be changed.

THINGS TO REMEMBER

- You can't take care of someone else if you can't take care of yourself.
- It's all about the moment; it's all about staying in the *now*.
- DSBT, holistic triage, the dimensions are important.
- Simple steps: I know it's overwhelming, but it *can* change.
- Breathing, music, soft lights, "me time"—come up with a name for this.
- It's not just about talking to you or someone else.
- It's about replacing the biopsychosocial paradigm with the cognitive-energy-movement paradigm.
- It's about breathing.
- It's about exhaling.
- It's about imagery.
- It's about nutrition.
- It's about hydration.
- It's about movement.
- It's about spirituality.
- It's about release.
- It's about caring for yourself…just like you care for someone else.
- It's about developing the "moment respites."

Hi Dr. Force,

The saga of dementia goes on and on. Attaching some notes of the past months since you met with us at the Parkinson Support Group in Warwick. I'm blown away by what some of those women in the group do in their caretaking tasks.

I received a book from a friend, *Meet Me Where I Am* by Mary Ann Drummond. The book was named for a writing in it I found poignant. It goes, "I'm no less creative, no less intelligent. I really am still me. My brain is simply wired a little differently now. Just a little jumbled and a bit mixed up. Don't discard me; I'm still here. But your world frightens me. Can you come to me? Meet me where I am, to laugh, to love, to share. Visit me here…and excuse the clutter…It's just a little jumbled and a bit mixed up."

Good luck with your writings.

M. J. (yes, anonymous to protect my husband's cool reputation as a hotshot)

M. J.'S STORY

My husband was diagnosed with mild cognitive impairment in early 2012 when I noticed continued confusion, agitation, and hallucinations in the evening. After in-depth cognitive testing, Joe was prescribed Aricept.

Within twenty-four hours he improved. In addition, Combigan, which is an eye drop for glaucoma, was stopped after I had looked up the side effects. Within twenty-four hours of discontinuing the eye drop, he again improved. An interim neurologist added Namenda XR after stating that my husband now had moderate cognitive impairment. He was leading a normal life, playing golf and driving his red Corvette convertible to the golf course daily. We attended a 13th Bomb Squadron reunion in New Orleans that year; walking aggravated Joe's right knee so much that he would need knee-replacement surgery in order to walk. We made another trip to Asheville, North Carolina to meet up with dear friends and with Joe's brother and wife. That was our last trip. After Joe's February 2013 knee surgery, he had confusion, disorientation, and hallucinations that abated after returning home. He rehabilitated from surgery very well and was back on the golf course. His game, formerly a four under par, had gone downhill, but he could still play though frustrated by that fact. Then came December 2013, when Joe had surgery for glaucoma. In the Doctor's absence, another Eye Physician convinced us that Joe must have surgery even though his pressure wasn't so high—not above seventeen. The doctor said it was the shape of the optic nerve. I stressed and discussed with the Doctor at great length my concern about Joe having surgery and anesthesia. Prior to surgery I spoke to three anesthesiologists regarding Joe's mild cognitive impairment (MCI). They told me that they typically add a narcotic to the anesthesia, and I told them *not* to, as Joe has adverse reactions to narcotics and other meds, which I had listed in writing to them. They administered Versed. Joe became animated and was hallucinating. They stopped the anesthesia; however, the doctor continued the surgery with local lidocaine and tetracaine. The doctor broke through the capsular; particles of cataract, which is removed if present when doing the bleb glaucoma surgery, went into the vitreous fluid. The doctor sent us to a retina specialist the next day. On and on it went. When the pressure measured zero in the operative eye, the doctor wanted us to see a doctor in Brooklyn. I took Joe to the specialists of our choice in New Jersey. He needed three surgeries just to correct the original. He had little effect from anesthesia each time. The anesthesiologist associated with the corrective surgeries commented to me that you never give Versed to a patient with cognitive impairment. The glaucoma specialist, after reviewing the prior doctor's records, stated he would not have done surgery—an unsolicited comment. Joe went into surgery driving, playing golf, fixing a cup of tea, and getting his own lunch. Besides the damage to the eyesight in the operative eye, it has affected his spatial perception and made his dementia so much worse.

In July of that year, Joe was diagnosed with Lewy body dementia, a dementia that later shows Parkinson's-like movement problems.

Joe has typical Parkinson's movement disorder, primarily in his gait. The shaking is minimal, however. The doctor changed Joe's meds simply by changing the time Joe takes them—in the evening instead of the morning. There was a huge difference—Joe was calmer in the day, more in the moment.

I feel it necessary to paint the picture of the diagnosis if only to alert others to avoid any surgeries and procedures that can be avoided and to be sure to get a second or third opinion should surgery be needed. Be sure the anesthesiologists are experienced in treating patients with dementia.

So began my journey as a caretaker.

My coping skills can wear thin. I pray daily for patience. It helps to put myself in his shoes. Patience and understanding of this man not being the same person is difficult.

Aging in place comes with a price: loss of privacy, poop nights, paranoia, nastiness, agitation, and all-around stress.

It helps to have grandchildren visit. However, even with a caregiver coming three times a week, it's difficult to get to some of the grandchildren's sporting events, plays, and so on. I need to start doing something routinely for myself. My walking and exercise routine has vanished. I vow to change that.

The most difficult, unmanageable parts are times such as when Joe had constipation and then trauma as a result of a visit to the ER. The dam broke at home. He had no way to understand that he had to go use the toilet. I spent hours running behind him from 2:00 a.m. on, cleaning up an unbelievable mess all over rugs and floors. I had to give him three showers. These things happen in the middle of the night. Another time, a similar situation arose with urination in the middle of the night; Joe hallucinated the toilet overflowing and so would not use it. He went on the carpeting and on the floor—another shower and cleanup at midnight. To get a caregiver at night for these, thus far few, unmanageable situations may not be my solution. We have a very small house. I would still be up and awake, helping. Another situation occurs when he gets belligerent and won't take pills and eye drops. I sometimes guess he's dehydrated if it's morning time, and in that state he also refuses to drink. It used to help to put our son on the phone to tell him to comply. That doesn't seem to work anymore.

I'm questioning my ability to keep him home as his dementia increases. I so did not want that to happen. He has lucid hours in the day and anxiety in the morning. I can't bear to think of him in a facility not getting the comfort he needs each day. I know that he would cease to be at all if I can't care for him at home. He looks to me, the assertive, controlling person, to solve an unsolvable problem. He realizes he's not right but doesn't understand the scope of it. Often he says he wishes he were dead.

I began these notes several months ago. Joe's condition has rapidly deteriorated. Though I'm still caring for him at home, we no longer can enjoy going out with friends for lunch or dinner. Eating is difficult for Joe spatially. He is not able to get the fork in the food and is having a hard time generally, taking the fun out of it.

Paranoia has set in to the point where he becomes incredibly difficult about the simplest things. Nighttime pee incidences have increased, and he needs to wear Depends. Most times, no matter how I approach it, he refuses. He claims he needs to call the FBI or 911 to say he's being kidnapped by a big blond lady—not me—always saying his wallet and money were stolen. Classic scenarios. He can get combative, shaking his fist, saying he knows I'm trying to kill him, but he'll kill me first. I'm very wary of situations and can move much faster than he can. I hesitate to tell the doctors, as they would likely have to act in some way, such as getting social services involved. I'm watching that situation closely and have visited assisted-living and long-term-care facilities. Given that I'm up with him four times a night because of his prostate problem, guiding him into the bathroom to use the toilet instead of the floor and getting him back in bed, I think he'd be kicked out of assisted living pretty quickly.

Last night, after two hours of trying to convince him to put on a Depend and get undressed for bed, he agreed. I must have tucked him in four times before he settled down. When I finally gave him a hug and a kiss, he said, "Hey, hey, none of that! I'm married." You've got to laugh sometimes, even when it's easier to cry.

I'm lonely for my husband—my lover, my friend, and my companion. I miss our conversations. I don't like giving up the role of wife for the role of caregiver 24/7.

I still, however, cannot bear the thought of him not living here, of him living in a facility. How cruel to spend possibly years and years of your life in a setting that is not home. I'm exhausted physically and emotionally. Lewy body dementia has robbed us of our life.

I hope that through the reading of this book, you now understand and appreciate how important caring for *you* is; it's so vital and important to you and to others.

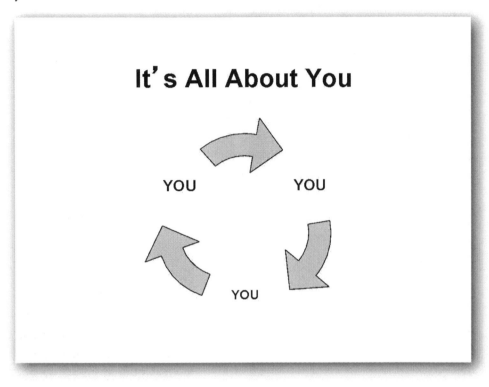

10

Nutrition and Exercise

It's so much more than food.

—Fifty-seven-year-old female caregiver

As I noted in the description of my practice intervention, dimensional solution-based treatment (DSBT), I place an emphasis on cognition, nutrition, and exercise. When clients come to see me in my practice, I tell them that this type of intervention (DSBT) may not be for everyone. However, if they have a commitment and a resolve to change, I encourage them to commit to examining and monitoring their nutritional intake and their exercise. I tell my clients, "You can't be eating fourteen bags of potato chips per day and drinking sixteen sodas and wonder why you might feel anxious and depressed. And hear me clearly: I am not suggesting that you only eat one meal per day or spend ten hours per day in the gym. Nutrition is important, and exercise and movement are vital, whether it be an enrollment in a gym or committing to walking daily or taking your dog on a long walk a couple of times per day." I typically refer my clients to three individuals that I think highly of: Louise Turino, RD, CDN, registered dietician and certified diabetes educator; Anne Keating Burger, RYT, certified yoga instructor; and Dallas Fuentes, MA, certified Pilates teacher. Below you will find their insightful comments as they relate to the importance of nutrition, exercise, and strength building.

The following are insights and an overview from Louise Turino, RD, CDN, registered dietician and certified diabetes educator. You can contact her at nardelli2@aol.com.

NUTRITION

Caring for another individual on a daily basis can be physically and emotionally exhausting. The additional stress you place on your body can be very taxing and may leave everyday life decisions more complicated. Stress has the potential to wreak havoc on the body and increase our risk for cancer and heart attack. This is when you need to make the transformation of not only caring for your loved one, but yourself.

The ultimate goal we need to achieve is how to sustain enough energy to get us through the day. In addition, how can we create the balance of a sound mind and a healthy body? It will take discipline and time to complete this task, but the results are priceless. As Aristotle said, "Let food be thy medicine, and medicine be thy food."

Those were the very words I embraced wholeheartedly after being faced with a case of pneumonia. I had the mentality of an eighteen-year-old—that my body can function like the everlasting Duracell battery, that my body could run on lack of sleep and poor nutrition without suffering any consequences. This came to a complete halt when my body responded to this self-inflicted abuse in a very negative way. I had lost a total of thirty-five pounds within a few weeks, and was faced with the possibility that my body might never recover. After that grueling recovery, I vowed to view my body as a temple.

My journey began with studying nutrition. I became a registered dietitian and wanted to live up to the expectation of being an expert in diet and nutrition. I wanted to educate as many people who were willing to listen on how to maintain equilibrium in the body and avoid the negative outcomes they might experience when they neglect their bodies. I wanted people to stop and ask themselves, "Am I really caring for myself?" You have to create a balance between caregiver and self. Because in the long run, you won't have the energy, and your own health may be jeopardized.

There were many occurrences in my own life when I found it difficult to keep my eyes from shutting. I needed to establish some type of healthy pattern with my sleep, food intake, and exercise. Sleep is essential for a person's health and well-being, according to the National Sleep Foundation (NSF). When you sleep it gives the body an opportunity to repair itself so that it can run smoothly. You should aim for at least seven to eight hours of sleep daily.

A large percentage of us skip meals. Over my years of counseling, sometimes the excuse is not having enough time in the day to eat. Food preparation and following a recipe can be difficult. Another excuse is that if they just don't eat as often, they will eventually lose weight. With food consumption, we're striving to try and provide the body with all the nutrients it needs in a given day. When you decrease your meal consumption, you also don't consume the adequate amounts of vitamins and minerals our bodies need in a day. Our emphasis should be on planning three meals daily, with nutrient-dense foods. Combine food items from the macronutrients: carbohydrate, protein, and fat. Nutrient deficiencies are linked to fatigue, poor mental function, and other health concerns.

- Many studies, of both adults and children, have shown that breakfast eaters tend to weigh less than breakfast skippers.
- Not only does it give you energy to start a new day, but also breakfast is linked to many health benefits, including weight control and improved performance.
- It's the simple sugars that you need to keep at a minimum. These are high-sugar food items that are easily absorbed in the bloodstream. They provide immediate energy but eventually, after a couple of hours, the body crashes. You want to avoid soda and other sugar-filled drinks.
- Carbohydrates impact blood sugar the most; protein and fat don't have as much of an impact. The type of carbohydrate you consume is very important. You want to include whole grains, fresh fruits, and vegetables. When consuming a carbohydrate at any

given meal, you also want to include a lean protein and a "good" fat. When you combine all three together, it slows the absorption of glucose in the bloodstream and prevents insulin spikes. It also prevents us from feeling hungry in a short period of time. A sample meal would be quinoa, lean turkey meat, and spinach.

- The basis of stabilizing blood sugars is to try and incorporate fiber with your meals. Fiber is the part of fruits and vegetables that can't be digested. Fiber helps move food through the digestive tract, helps lower cholesterol, and prevents constipation. Most whole grains are a good source of fiber. Fiber also helps the food you ingest stay in the stomach longer. This is satiety, the feeling of fullness after eating a meal. It helps suppresses the urge to eat for a period of time after a meal. Women need to consume, on average, twenty-eight grams of fiber daily, and men need to consume thirty-eight grams per day, according to the Institute of Medicine.

- There are two broad types of fiber: soluble and insoluble. Soluble fiber dissolves in water. It changes as it goes through the digestive tract, where it is fermented by bacteria. As it absorbs water it becomes gelatinous. Insoluble fiber does not dissolve in water. As it goes through the digestive tract it does not change its form.

WAYS TO INCLUDE FRUITS AND VEGETABLES
Keep it simple. Here are some examples:

- Add frozen or fresh berries to your oatmeal.
- Put mushrooms, onion, spinach, pineapple, or peppers on your pizza.
- Add peanut butter to your apple.
- Include cucumbers, avocado, carrots, and pear in salads.

Everyone's perception of a serving size is very different. I can vouch for this in the decades of providing medical nutrition. When an individual is asked how much of an item do he or she consumes, I get such varied answers. What we conceive to be a bowl can be significantly different from how another person views a bowl. According to the National Institutes of Health, a *portion* is how much food you choose to eat at one time, whether in a restaurant, from a package, or in your own kitchen. A *serving size* is a specific amount of food or drink, such as a cup of yogurt or a slice of bread.

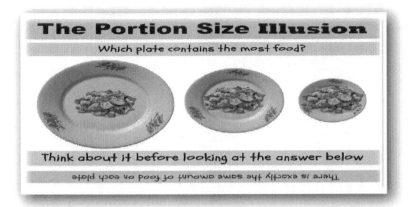

That's why it's extremely important to observe food labels for serving sizes. Many individuals will regularly skip meals because they hold the false idea that they will eat fewer calories throughout the day. Others skip meals because they just don't have enough time to make something. Others skip regularly, thinking they will take in fewer total calories and lose weight.

SUPERFOODS

While many foods are important for heart health, a few are superfoods with extra power to protect your heart. These superfoods help to fight heart disease because they contain one or more of the following ingredients:

- **Antioxidants:** Antioxidants help to eliminate harmful free radicals called *oxidants* that result from the body's natural oxidation process. Free radicals are believed to contribute to a host of health problems including heart disease, diabetes, and cancer. Antioxidants also might help to boost the immune system.
- **Anti-inflammatories:** In recent years, studies have shown that chronic inflammation is a risk factor for heart disease as well as stroke, diabetes, and even some cancers.
- **Omega-3 fatty acids:** Studies have shown that these unsaturated fatty acids can be powerful contributors to heart health, possibly by reducing inflammation. They also appear to reduce blood clots that can cause strokes and might slow cognitive problems such as Alzheimer's disease and age-related cognitive deterioration.

- **Monounsaturated and polyunsaturated fats:** In contrast to saturated fats and trans fats, or the "bad" fats, monounsaturated and polyunsaturated fats are "good" fats that can help to reduce LDL or bad cholesterol in the blood and reduce the risk of heart attack and stroke. In addition, monounsaturated fats usually contain vitamin E, an antioxidant.

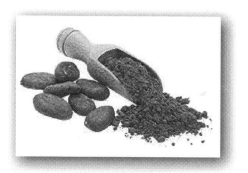

- **Cocoa:** Cocoa contains hundreds of compounds that boost endorphins and serotonin, two of the best-known chemicals responsible for making us happy. It's known for its flavonoids, chemicals found naturally in plants that may help fight a wide array of conditions including diabetes, stroke, and heart disease

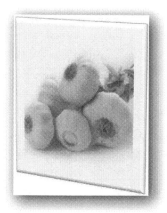

- **Garlic:** Garlic has the sulfur compound allicin, an amino acid. Allicin is not present in whole garlic, but it is formed instantly when garlic is crushed, chewed, or cut.

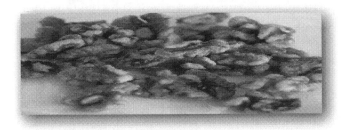

- **Walnuts:** Walnuts contain alpha-Linoleic acid, an omega-3 fatty acid. Walnuts have been shown to lower cholesterol and have been associated with better heart health. They are packed with antioxidants and also contain vitamin E, folic acid, zinc, and protein. If you don't like walnuts, try chia seeds. Yes, the ones from the Chia Pet commercials—these seeds are high in omega-3 fatty acids.

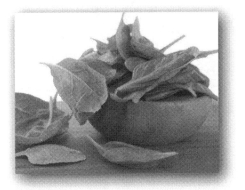

- **Spinach:** Spinach is filled with antioxidants including vitamin C and beta-carotene as well as lutein and zeaxanthin. One cup of fresh spinach leaves also provides almost double the daily requirement for vitamin K, which plays an important role in cardiovascular and bone health. And of course you can't forget that spinach is a great vegetarian source of iron, which keeps your hair and nails strong and healthy. Use fresh spinach leaves as a base for salad, or sauté them and add them to an omelet. Spinach also has antioxidants that fight cancer and inflammation. Researchers have identified more than a dozen different flavonoid compounds in spinach that function as anti-inflammatory and anticancer agents.

EXERCISE

Move a muscle, change a thought.

—ALCOHOLICS ANONYMOUS

The following are insights and an overview from Anne Keating Burger, RYT, certified yoga instructor. You can contact her at keatinga@hotmail.com.

THE BENEFITS OF EXERCISE IN RECOVERY

Many individuals who assume the role of caregiver neglect important components of daily health, wreaking havoc on both emotional and physical well-being. It is important to repair the psychological and physical damage of chemical dependency as well as the damaged mind-body connection.

- Exercise relieves and reduces stress. Exercise has been shown to alleviate both physical and psychological stress. Moving your body alleviates this tension and allows you to get rid of any negative emotions you have been keeping in. Focused exercise uses both physical and emotional energy that might otherwise find unhealthy ways of escaping.
- Exercising naturally and positively alters your brain chemistry. When you exercise, your body releases endorphins, which create a natural high. However, stress and anxiety causes an imbalance that interferes with a person's ability to feel pleasure, happiness, and satisfaction. Dedicated physical activity during your caregiving day will help reintroduce natural levels of endorphins in your system. This not only helps you feel better but also teaches your body that it is capable of regulating its own brain chemistry and mood in healthy, natural ways.
- "Exercise is meditation in motion." The Mayo Clinic has described exercise as "meditation in motion," meaning that by concentrating on the physical, we can experience the psychological and emotional

benefits of meditation. Through movement, we can refocus our thoughts on our own well-being and forget, at least briefly, all that is going on in our lives.

- Exercise improves your outlook. Those who exercise regularly report increased feelings of self-confidence and optimism and reduced feelings of depression and anxiety. This is in part to do with the body regulating and calibrating itself during exercise, but it also has to do with feelings of accomplishment, pride, and self-worth as you see your body transform and your goals reached. As you reach certain benchmarks, you feel more accomplished, and this reinforces the goal of continued sobriety as attainable. Regular exercise also fosters improved sleep, greater energy, and enhanced feelings of well-being.

BENEFITS OF YOGA IN RECOVERY

Replace artificial highs for natural ones. Caregivers are used to overindulging in lots of things: eating too much, drinking and taking drugs, gossiping too much, shopping too much, smoking too much, and so on. These overindulgences fill the emptiness on the inside, using external things to fill the inside holes. Yoga, specifically meditation, teaches us to draw our awareness away from these external stimuli, detach from our senses, and direct our attention inward. Yoga is also known to help individuals eliminate reactiveness, find community, develop control of mind, increase control over stress and anxiety levels, and repair the nervous system.

The following are insights and an overview from Dallas Fuentes, MA, certified Pilates teacher. Contact her at www.perfectpartspilates.com/dallas-fuentes.

STRENGTH BUILDING (PILATES)

Poise, graceful movement, and greater spatial awareness are the natural outcomes of the beginning stages of Pilates work. A logical progression of corrective exercises, which address structural flaws causing muscular and joint pain, postural strain, stiffness, and loss of muscle tone, will be employed. Working to strengthen the supportive musculature in the center of the body lays the foundation for creating lasting structural change, thereby also influencing self-concept. The novel exercises performed in Pilates offer a great range that is developed for each person on an individualized basis. The routines are creative, challenging, and mind engaging. The six principles of the Pilates method (centering, control, concentration, precision, flow, and breath) will be incorporated into each individual's practice.

The overall goal of nutrition, exercise, and strength building is twofold: to stop the destructive patterns and to develop support strategies to maintain long-term recovery. With the incorporation of healthy nutrition and exercise practices into the daily life of the individual, tension and stress reduction are measureable and productive outcomes, thereby enhancing positive outlook and increased self-esteem.

11

Summary Points

"It is all about you"—a familiar and important theme. You have a responsibility or role to be present for someone. Either you have stepped up and taken on the domains of this role, or it has been thrust upon you—or a combination of the two. However you have arrived here in this part of your life, you are here. Now the focus, energy, and work are to help you move through this area.

Some individuals put their own life on hold. Others "build a life within a life"; they look at this caregiver role as an opportunity to rediscover themselves. Some caregivers will see a new life in this role, and some caregivers will watch their life wash away. However movement occurs, I have one promise: there will be a time that this role will cease, and then what's next? It's an interesting question, with a variety of outcomes as unique as the person.

Caregiving is an inside job—and it is all about you!

In essence, if you want to survive caregiving—act like you do!

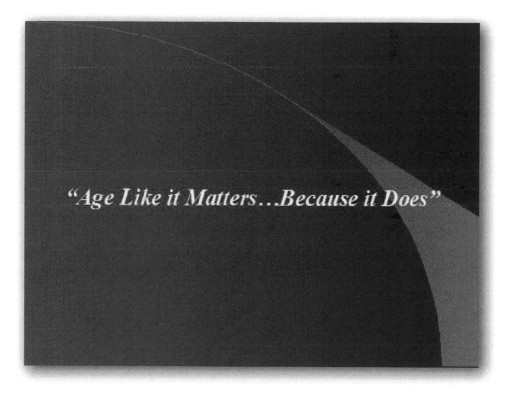

12

Resource Section

This section provides connections to resources, services, and programs on the national, state, and local level.

Disclaimer: Please note that this information is not an endorsement of a particular resource, service, or program. You, as the caregiver, relating to your own life and situation, will decide on your own as to the merit and value of these entities.

Here is additional evidence and support—you are not alone.

The following is a guide of information and services for the elderly, their families, or other care providers. It includes information and Internet links to services and programs. This list contains only a sample of the resources that are available on the Internet for the elderly.

AMERICAN ASSOCIATION OF RETIRED PEOPLE, HTTP://WWW.AARP.ORG/

AARP is a nonprofit, nonpartisan membership organization for people fifty and over. They provide information and resources; advocate on legislative, consumer, and legal issues; assist members to serve their communities; and offer a wide range of unique benefits, special products, and services for their members. These benefits include the www.aarp.org, *Modern Maturity* and *My Generation* magazines, and the monthly *AARP Bulletin*. Active in every state, the District of Columbia, Puerto Rico, and the US Virgin

Islands, AARP celebrates the attitude that age is just a number, and life is what you make of it.

ADMINISTRATION ON AGING (AOA), WWW.AOA.GOV

The Administration on Aging (AOA) is the principal agency of the US Department of Health and Human Services designated to carry out the provisions of the Older Americans Act of 1965 (OAA) as amended (42 US Code 3001). The OAA promotes the well-being of older individuals by providing services and programs designed to help them live independently in their homes and communities. The act also empowers the federal government to distribute funds to the states for supportive services for individuals over the age of sixty. The resource directory is intended to serve a wide audience including older people and their families, health and legal professionals, social-service providers, librarians, researchers, and others with an interest in the field of aging. The directory contains names, addresses, phone numbers, and fax numbers of organizations that provide information and other resources on matters relating to the needs of older persons. Inclusion in the directory does not imply an endorsement or recommendation by NIA or AoA.

ALZHEIMER'S ASSOCIATION, HTTP://WWW.ALZ.ORG

The Alzheimer's Association, a national network of chapters, is the largest national voluntary health organization committed to finding a cure for Alzheimer's and helping those affected by the disease. The Alzheimer's Association is your source for information, support, and assistance on issues related to early onset Alzheimer's and Alzheimer's disease.

AGEPLAN INC., HTTP://WWW.AGEPLAN.COM

AgePlan, a provider of resources, services, and solutions in the field of aging, disability, and lifespan development was founded in 2004. AgePlan Inc. is a *leading nationwide provider* of educational and consulting services to agencies, businesses, communities, families, and individuals, with regard to aging and disability.

THE AMERICAN FEDERATION OF AGING RESEARCH, HTTP://WWW.AFAR.ORG/

This is America's leading private organization, supporting new investigators conducting biomedical aging research. The fact sheets are designed for professionals in the field of aging. Each fact sheet includes an overview of the subject and details related to Administration on Aging initiatives.

THE JOHN A. HARTFORD FOUNDATION INSTITUTE FOR GERIATRIC NURSING, HTTP://WWW.JHARTFOUND.ORG/

The Hartford Institute for Geriatric Nursing seeks to shape the quality of health care for older Americans by promoting the highest level of geriatric competence in all nurses. By raising the standards of nursing care, the Hartford Institute aims to ensure that people age with optimal function, comfort, and dignity.

HEALTHFINDER, HTTP://WWW.HEALTHFINDER.GOV

Healthfinder is a free guide to reliable consumer health and human services information, developed by the US Department of Health and Human Services. Healthfinder can lead you to selected online publications, clearinghouses, databases, websites, and support and self-help groups, as well as government agencies and not-for-profit organizations that produce reliable information for the public.

THE HUFFINGTON CENTER ON AGING, HTTP://WWW.HCOA.ORG/

This is one of the most advanced aging research programs in the country. Especially prominent are their programs in cell and molecular biology of aging, cardiovascular disease, ethics, and outcomes research. Research geriatricians and gerontologists are trained through an NIA-funded aging-research training grant and an approved geriatrics fellowship program that offers two additional years of research training for those interested in academic research careers. Research enrichment, including opportunities to visit laboratories in this country and abroad, is afforded by the generosity of several foundations.

INSTITUTE FOR HEALTH AND AGING, HTTP://WWW.NURSEWEB.UCSF.EDU/IHA/

This site aims to optimize the health and aging of individuals' community and society through research, education, and public service in the social, behavioral, and policy sciences.

JOINT COMMISSION ON ACCREDITATION OF HEALTHCARE ORGANIZATIONS, HTTP://WWW.JCAHO.ORG/

JCAHO is continuously improving the safety and quality of care provided to the public through the provision of healthcare accreditation and related services that support performance improvement in health-care organizations.

NATIONAL COUNCIL ON AGING (NCOA), WWW.NCOA.ORG

The NCOA provides innovative support and assistance programs for senior centers, Area Agencies on Aging, adult day facilities, and other local service organizations in the field of aging. Their advocacy efforts have resulted in significant legislative victories for older Americans on Capitol Hill. NCOA's workforce division has exceeded its goals for coordinating the hiring of low-income older Americans. They continue to foster innovations that improve the quality of services for older people.

NATIONAL HEALTH INFORMATION CENTER (NHIC), HTTP://WWW.HEALTH.GOV/NHIC/

The National Health Information Center (NHIC) is a health information referral service. NHIC puts health professionals and consumers who have health questions in touch with those organizations that are best able to provide answers.

NATIONAL INSTITUTE ON AGING (NIA), HTTPS://WWW.NIA.NIH.GOV/

The NIA's mission is to improve the health and well-being of older Americans through research and specifically to support and conduct high-quality research on the aging process, age-related diseases, and special problems and needs of the aged.

NATIONAL INSTITUTES OF HEALTH (NIH): HTTP://WWW.NIH.GOV/

The NIH's mission is to uncover new knowledge that will lead to better health for everyone. The NIH works toward that mission by conducting research in its own laboratories; supporting the research of nonfederal scientists in universities, medical schools, hospitals, and research institutions throughout the country and abroad; helping in the training of research investigators; and fostering communication of medical information.

NATIONAL LIBRARY OF MEDICINE, HTTP://WWW.NLM.NIH.GOV/

Every significant program of the library is represented, from medical history to biotechnology. They hope that the resources of the world's largest biomedical library will find even wider useful applications around the nation and around the world.

RETIREMENT RESEARCH FOUNDATION, HTTP://WWW.RRF.ORG

For more than thirty years, RRF has been at the forefront of efforts to meet the ever-changing needs of older Americans. They have invested more than $115 million to help build a network of innovative and skilled individuals and institutions committed to addressing aging and retirement issues.

ROBERT WOOD JOHNSON FOUNDATION, HTTP://WWW.RWJF.ORG/MAIN.HTML

The Robert Wood Johnson Foundation was established as a national philanthropy in 1972, and today it is the largest US foundation devoted to improving the health and health care of all Americans.

SOCIAL SECURITY ADMINISTRATION, HTTP://WWW.SSA.GOV/

This website provides an online directory plus information on benefits, services for businesses, research data, financing, planning and budgets, Social Security laws, and reporting fraud.

THE GERONTOLOGICAL SOCIETY OF AMERICA, HTTP://WWW.GERON.ORG/

The Gerontological Society of America promotes the conduct of multi- and interdisciplinary research in aging by expanding and improving the quality of gerontological research and by increasing its funding resources. It also disseminates gerontological research knowledge to researchers, practitioners, and decision and opinion makers.

AGING AND ALCOHOL, HTTP://PUBS.NIAAA.NIH.GOV/PUBLICATIONS/AA40.HTM

Anyone at any age can have a drinking problem. Great Uncle George might have always been a heavy drinker, but his family might find that as he gets older, the problems get worse. Grandma Betty may have been a teetotaler all her life, just taking a drink to help her sleep after her husband died. Now she needs a couple of drinks to get through the day. Drinking problems in older people are often neglected by families, doctors, and the public.

THE NATIONAL ORGANIZATION OF ADULT ADDICTIONS AND RECOVERY INC. (NOAAR), HTTP:WWW.NOAAR.ORG

The National Organization for Adult Addictions and Recovery (NOAAR) mission is to raise awareness and to treat and prevent addictions in adults, midlife, and beyond. They provide clinical expertise, training, and consultative services to individuals, family members, professionals, and organizations. Goals for membership and the general population are achieved through personal consultations, conferences, educational modules, and web-based technologies.

INSTITUTE ON AGING, HTTP://WWW.MED.UPENN.EDU/AGING/
The Institute on Aging's intent is to improve the physiological, psychological, and social well-being of older persons through state-of-the-art interdisciplinary research, education, and clinical services.

CLINICALTRIALS.GOV, HTTP://WWW.CLINICALTRIALS.GOV
A service of the US National Institutes of Health, ClinicalTrials.gov is a registry and results database of publicly and privately supported clinical studies of human participants conducted around the world. Learn more about clinical studies and about this site, including relevant history, policies, and laws.

(Please use the following pages as an opportunity to reflect, take notes, write questions, develop goals and daily strategies, record feelings...or whatever else you may find of value and useful in guiding your caregiving day.)

NOTES/THOUGHTS/REFLECTIONS/ACTIONS

NOTES/THOUGHTS/REFLECTIONS/ACTIONS

NOTES/THOUGHTS/REFLECTIONS/ACTIONS

NOTES/THOUGHTS/REFLECTIONS/ACTIONS

_____

_____

_____

_____

_____

_____

_____

_____

_____

_____

_____

_____

_____

_____

_____

_____

_____

_____

_____

_____

_____

_____

_____

_____

_____

_____

_____

_____

_____

_____

NOTES/THOUGHTS/REFLECTIONS/ACTIONS

NOTES/THOUGHTS/REFLECTIONS/ACTIONS

_____

_____

_____

_____

_____

_____

_____

_____

_____

_____

_____

_____

_____

_____

_____

_____

_____

_____

_____

_____

_____

_____

_____

_____

_____

_____

_____

NOTES/THOUGHTS/REFLECTIONS/ACTIONS

NOTES/THOUGHTS/REFLECTIONS/ACTIONS

NOTES/THOUGHTS/REFLECTIONS/ACTIONS

NOTES/THOUGHTS/REFLECTIONS/ACTIONS

_____

_____

_____

_____

_____

_____

_____

_____

_____

_____

_____

_____

_____

_____

_____

_____

_____

_____

_____

_____

_____

_____

_____

_____

_____

_____

_____

_____

_____

_____

_____

NOTES/THOUGHTS/REFLECTIONS/ACTIONS

NOTES/THOUGHTS/REFLECTIONS/ACTIONS

NOTES/THOUGHTS/REFLECTIONS/ACTIONS

NOTES/THOUGHTS/REFLECTIONS/ACTIONS

NOTES/THOUGHTS/REFLECTIONS/ACTIONS

About the Author

Lawrence T. Force, PhD, LCSW-R, NBCCH

Dr. Lawrence T. Force, a gerontologist, has worked in the field of aging and disabilities for over thirty years as a practitioner, academician, administrator, and researcher in both the public and private sector. Dr. Force is the founder and CEO of AgePlan, a national advocacy and training organization and has recently helped launch the National Organization of Adult Addictions and Recovery (NOAAR), whose mission is to raise awareness and treat and prevent addictions in adults, those in midlife, and those beyond. He is a professor of psychology at Mount Saint Mary College and the director of the Center on Aging and Policy. Dr. Force is a nationally recognized leader in the area of end-of-life care for people with developmental disabilities and coauthor of *Gerontology: An Interactive Text* and *End-of-Life Care: A Guide for Supporting Older People with Intellectual Disabilities and Their Families*. He has authored and collaborated on books, articles, chapters, monographs, and technical reports that address topics such as developmental models of aging, caregiving, addictions across the lifespan, lifelong disabilities, and naturally occurring living communities (NOLCs). Dr. Force was sponsored as a summer institute fellow at the National Institute on Aging (NIA) and the RAND Corporation and was funded as a principal investigator (PI) on a National Institute of Health (NIH) grant conducting a nationwide study of the Area Agencies on Aging (AAAs). He has presented his work at national and international conferences. Dr. Force is a licensed clinical social worker (LCSW-R) and a National Board Certified Clinical Hypnotherapist (NBCCH)